Chambers

classical roots
for medics

Chambers

Chambers

An imprint of Chambers Harrap Publishers Ltd
7 Hopetoun Crescent
Edinburgh
EH7 4AY

© Chambers Harrap Publishers Ltd 2007

First published by Chambers Harrap Publishers Ltd 2007

A CIP catalogue record for this book is available from the British Library.

ISBN-13: 978 0550 10349 9

Designed and typeset by Chambers Harrap Publishers Ltd, Edinburgh
Printed by Clays Ltd, St Ives plc

Contributors

Editor
Katie Brooks

Lexicographer
Donald Watt

Prepress
Andrew Butterworth

Publishing Manager
Camilla Rockwood

The editor would like to thank the following people for their invaluable comments on the manuscript:

Jamie Davies, Professor in Experimental Anatomy at the University of Edinburgh;

Dr Edward Duvall, Senior Lecturer at the University of Edinburgh and Honorary Consultant in Cytopathology at the Royal Infirmary of Edinburgh.

Contents

Introduction

Chambers Classical Roots for Medics has been specifically designed for people who need to understand medical terminology and become familiar with it, including medical students and students of other subjects allied to medicine. The sheer volume of medical vocabulary can in itself be extremely daunting to students, and the constituent words can seem very complicated. This is mainly because many medical terms come from either Greek or Latin, languages that would once have been familiar to students but are now studied less and less frequently.

This book aims to demystify medical terminology by showing how many words can be broken down into common 'building blocks' that come from Greek or Latin roots. Understanding the meaning of each of these components allows the meaning of whole words to be deduced. By becoming familiar with a relatively small number of these 'building blocks', students can therefore reduce the need for rote learning of vast numbers of words and are better equipped to cope with unfamiliar terms.

The main part of the book contains entries giving the derivation and meaning of each word or combining form. Plentiful examples of usage are also provided where appropriate. Extensive cross-referencing allows the reader to find related words, terms with opposite meanings, and equivalent terms from the two languages; terms that might easily be confused are also indicated. Although the purpose of *Chambers Classical Roots for Medics* is definitely not to teach written or spoken Latin or Greek, a brief appendix provides some basic information on forming plurals and making adjectives agree with nouns, ensuring that the book provides a practical guide to understanding and using medical vocabulary.

Note regarding transliteration

All Greek words that occur within the text have been represented using the Roman alphabet, so that no knowledge of the Greek alphabet is required. In transliterating these words we have attempted to make the spelling of the Greek roots as similar as possible to the English derivations. For this reason, the Greek character υ (upsilon) is represented by the letter 'y' where it occurs after a consonant (as in 'hypo-') but by the letter 'u' where it occurs after a vowel (as in 'neuro-'). Similarly, the Greek character χ (chi) is represented by 'ch' rather than by 'kh' (as in 'brachy-'). We trust that any scholars of Greek will be forgiving on this point.

The Greek characters ε (epsilon) and η (eta) are both represented by the letter 'e', but by a 'short' and a 'long' form respectively. The short 'e' has no mark, and is pronounced as in the English word 'men'. The long 'e' has a macron (long bar) over it (ē), and is pronounced as in the English word 'be'. Similarly, the Greek characters o (omicron) and ω (omega) are represented by the short and long forms of the letter 'o' respectively. The short 'o' has no mark, and is pronounced as in the English word 'got'. The long 'o' has a macron over it (ō), and is pronounced as in the English word 'go'.

How to use this book

Structure of entries

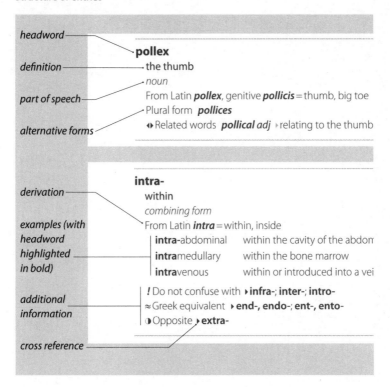

headword	**pollex**
definition	the thumb
part of speech	*noun*
	From Latin **pollex**, genitive **pollicis** = thumb, big toe
	Plural form **pollices**
alternative forms	◆ Related words **pollical** *adj* ▸ relating to the thumb

	intra-	
derivation	within	
	combining form	
examples (with headword highlighted in bold)	From Latin **intra** = within, inside	
	intra-abdominal	within the cavity of the abdom
	intramedullary	within the bone marrow
	intravenous	within or introduced into a vei
additional information	*!* Do not confuse with ▸ **infra-**; **inter-**; **intro-**	
	≈ Greek equivalent ▸ **end-, endo-; ent-, ento-**	
	◐ Opposite ▸ **extra-**	
cross reference		

Symbols

! indicates a term that might be confused with the headword
≈ indicates the Greek equivalent of a Latin headword, or vice versa.
◐ indicates a term with the opposite meaning to the headword
◆ indicates a term related to the headword

Abbreviations

adj	adjective	*med*	medicine
adv	adverb	*n*	noun
anat	anatomy	*pathol*	pathology
biochem	biochemistry	*psych*	psychiatry
dent	dentistry	*psychol*	psychology
genet	genetics	*vet med*	vetinary medicine

Aa

a-, an-
   not, without
   combining form
   From Greek **a-** = not, without
afebrile	not feverish
anaemia	a lack of red blood cells or haemoglobin
anorexia	a lack of appetite
aphasia	the inability to generate or understand speech
asymptomatic	having no symptoms

   ! Do not confuse with ▸**ana-**; **ano-**

---

ab-
   away, from
   combining form
   From Latin **ab** = away, from
abduction	the movement of a body part away from the midline of the body
ablation	the surgical removal of an organ or body tissue

   ≈ Greek equivalent ▸**apo-**

---

acinus
   a small sac, such as the air sacs of the lungs or the secretory sacs of glands
   noun
   From Latin **acinus** = grape, berry
   Plural form **acini**
   ◆ Related words **acinar** *adj* ▸relating to an acinus or acini

---

acro-
   denoting a tip, extremity, height
   combining form
   From Greek **akron** = highest point, extremity
acrocyanosis	bluish discoloration of the hands and feet
acromegaly	excessive growth of the hands, feet and face
acrophobia	a pathological fear of heights

---

actin-, actino-
   denoting rays; denoting radiation
   combining form
   From Greek **aktis**, genitive **aktinos** = ray

| ***Actino***bacillus | a genus of bacteria, species of which tend to form branched filaments |
| **actino**therapy | treatment involving exposure to electromagnetic radiation, especially ultraviolet light or X-rays |

ad-
towards, near, next to
combining form
From Latin ***ad*** = towards, near, next to

| **ad**duction | the movement of a body part towards the midline of the body |
| **ad**renal | next to the kidneys |

aden-, adeno-
denoting a gland
combining form
From Greek ***adēn*** = gland

adenitis	inflammation of a gland or glands
adenocarcinoma	a malignant tumour showing glandular differentiation
adenoma	a benign tumour in a gland or with a structure similar to that of a gland

adipo-
denoting fat
combining form
From Latin ***adeps***, genitive ***adipis*** = fat

| **adipo**cere | a fatty, waxy substance resulting from the decomposition of dead bodies in moist conditions |
| **adipo**cyte | a cell that stores fat |

≈ Greek equivalent ▸ **lip-, lipo-**; **pimel-, pimelo-**; **steat-, steato-**

adipose
fatty
adjective
From modern Latin ***adiposus*** = fatty, from Latin ***adeps***, genitive ***adipis*** = fat

| **adipose** tissue | body tissue used for storing fat |

adventitious
acquired or arising in a different location; relating to the tunica adventitia, the outermost layer of the wall of an organ or vessel
adjective
From Latin ***adventicius*** = extraneous

-aemia
denoting blood or the presence of a substance in the blood
combining form
From Greek *-aimia*, from **haima** = blood

an**aemia**	a lack of red blood cells or haemoglobin
hyperglyc**aemia**	an excessively high blood sugar level
leuk**aemia**	a cancerous disease in which too many white blood cells accumulate in the body
septic**aemia**	blood poisoning caused by bacteria or other micro-organisms

aer-, aero-
denoting air
combining form
From Greek *aēr* = air

aeration	the introduction of oxygen into the blood through respiration
aerophagia	the swallowing of air

aerobic
requiring oxygen to live and grow; denoting oxygen consumption
adjective
From Greek *aēr* = air + **bios** = life

aerobic bacteria	bacteria that require oxygen to live and grow
aerobic exercise	exercise that increases oxygen consumption and causes a sustained increase in heart rate and breathing
aerobic respiration	the process by which cells use oxygen to produce energy required for life

-aesthesia
denoting sensation or sensing
combining form
From Greek *aisthēsis* = sensation

an**aesthesia**	the loss of sensation of pain
hyper**aesthesia**	excessive sensitivity to physical sensations
kin**aesthesia**	the sensing of the position and movement of body parts

-aesthetic
denoting sensation or sensing
combining form
From Greek *aisthēsis* = sensation

an**aesthetic**	relating to or producing the loss of sensation of pain

hyper**aesthetic**	excessively sensitive to physical sensations
kin**aesthetic**	relating to the sensing of the position and movement of body parts

afferent

conveying towards a body part or organ

adjective

From Latin **afferens**, genitive **afferentis** = carrying towards, from **ad** = towards and **ferre** = to carry

afferent nerve	a nerve that conveys impulses to the brain or spinal cord

◑ Opposite ▸ **efferent**

-affin

denoting affinity or attraction

combining form

From Latin **affinis** = neighbouring, from **ad** = towards or near and **finis** = a boundary

argent**affin**	having an affinity for silver, said of tissues that bind silver salts
chrom**affin**	having an affinity for chromium, said of tissues that bind chromium salts

≈ Greek equivalent ▸ **-philic**

-agogue

denoting a substance that causes another specified substance to be secreted

combining form

From Greek **agōgos** = leading, from **agein** = to lead

chol**agogue**	a substance that causes bile to flow from the gall bladder into the duodenum
dacry**agogue**	a substance that causes the lachrymal glands to secrete tears
galact**agogue**	a substance that promotes secretion of milk

ala

a flat winglike structure

noun

From Latin **ala** = wing

Plural form **alae**

nasal **ala**	the winglike piece of cartilage forming the outer side of a nostril

-algesia

denoting sensitivity to pain

combining form

From Greek **algēsis** = sense of pain

   an**algesia**   a lack of sensitivity to pain

◆ Related words **-algesic** *adj* ▸relating to sensitivity to pain

-algia

denoting pain in a particular part of the body

combining form

From Greek **algos** = pain

   cephal**algia**   headache

   my**algia**   pain in a muscle

   neur**algia**   pain in a nerve

◆ Related words **-algic** *adj* ▸relating to pain in a particular part of the body

allo-

other, different

combining form

From Greek **allos** = other

   allograft   a tissue graft from a genetically different donor

   allopathy   the treatment of disease by inducing an effect that is
                     different from those caused by the disease

◖ Opposite ▸**homeo-**

alveolus

a small cavity or sac-like structure

noun

From Latin **alveolus** = small pit, from Latin **alveus** = a hollow

Plural form **alveoli**

   dental **alveolus**   a tooth socket

   pulmonary   one of the small thin-walled sacs in the lung
     alveolus   through which gaseous exchange takes place with the
                   pulmonary capillaries

◆ Related words **alveolar** *adj* ▸relating to a small cavity or sac-like structure

amnio-

denoting the amnion (innermost membrane) enveloping an embryo

combining form

From Greek **amnion** = caul (the membrane that covers a newborn mammal at birth)

amniocentesis	the puncturing of the amnion with a hollow needle to take a sample of the fluid surrounding an embryo
amnioscopy	an examination of the interior of the amnion with a viewing instrument
amniotomy	the cutting of the amnion to induce labour

amnion

the innermost membrane enveloping an embryo
noun
From Greek ***amnion*** = caul (the membrane that covers a newborn mammal at birth)
Plural form **amnia** (or **amnions**)
◆ Related words **amniotic** *adj* ▸relating to the amnion

amphi-

both, on both sides
combining form
From Greek ***amphi*** = on both sides

| **amphi**arthrosis | a joint that allows only slight movement in either direction |

an- see ▸ a-, an-

ana-

up
combining form
From Greek ***ana*** = up

anabolic steroids	steroids used to increase the build-up of body tissue such as muscle
analeptic	a drug used to stimulate the central nervous system
anatomy	the science of the structure of the human body learned by cutting it up

! Do not confuse with ▸ **a-, an-**; **ano-**
◑ Opposite ▸ **cat-, cata-**

anal see ▸ anus

andro-

denoting man, male
combining form
From Greek ***anēr***, genitive ***andros*** = man

androgen   a male sex hormone

andrology   the study of functions and diseases specific to males

◑ Opposite ▸ **gyn-, gynaeco-, gyno-**

---

angi-, angio-
denoting a blood or lymph vessel
combining form
From Greek ***angeion*** = vessel

angiography the X-raying of blood vessels

angioma   a tumour consisting mainly of blood vessels (also
        haemangioma) or lymph vessels (also *lymphangioma*)

angioplasty   a method of restoring a blocked or narrowed blood
        vessel to its original shape

---

anis-, aniso-
denoting unequal
combining form
From Greek ***anisos*** = unequal, from ***a-*** = not and ***isos*** = equal

anisomelia   a difference in the lengths of paired limbs

anisopia   a difference in vision between the eyes

---

ano-
denoting the anus
combining form
From Latin ***anus*** = anus

anogenital   relating to the anus and the genitals

anorectal   relating to the anus and the rectum

! Do not confuse with ▸ **a-, an-; ana-**
≈ Latin equivalent ▸ **proct-, procto-**

---

ante-
before, forwards
combining form
From Latin ***ante*** = before, forwards

anteflexion   the bending forwards of an organ, especially the uterus

antenatal   before birth

antepartum   before labour

! Do not confuse with ▸ **anti-**
≈ Greek equivalent ▸ **pro-**
◑ Opposite ▸ **post-**

anterior

nearer to the front of the human body or to the front of a part of the human body

adjective

From Latin ***anterior*** = front

anterior cruciate ligament	the front ligament of a pair of ligaments that cross each other in the knee

◑ Opposite ▸ **posterior**

anti-

acting against, preventing, counteracting; opposite, reverse

combining form

From Greek ***anti*** = against

antiarrhythmic	counteracting an abnormal heartbeat
antibacterial	preventing bacterial infection
anticoagulant	preventing blood from clotting
antidepressant	a drug used to counteract depression
antiperistalsis	contraction of the intestine in the opposite direction to normal

! Do not confuse with ▸ **ante-**

≈ Latin equivalent ▸ **contra-**

antrum

a natural cavity, especially in a bone

noun

From Latin ***antrum*** = cave

Plural form **antra**

mastoid **antrum**	a cavity in the mastoid bone behind the ear

◆ Related words **antral** *adj* ▸relating to a natural cavity, especially in a bone

anus

the opening at the end of the alimentary canal through which solid waste is eliminated

noun

From Latin ***anus*** = anus

◆ Related words **anal** *adj* ▸relating to the anus

apex

the tip of an organ (*med*); the root tip of a tooth (*dent*)

noun

From Latin ***apex***, genitive ***apicis*** = top, tip

Plural form **apices** (or **apexes**)

◆ Related words **apical** *adj* ▸relating to the tip of an organ or to the root tip of a tooth

---

apo-
from, away from
combining form
From Greek ***apo*** = from, away from

apomorphine	an alkaloid derived from morphine used as an emetic, an expectorant and in the treatment of Parkinson's disease
apophysis	an outgrowth from a bone
apoptosis	the natural destruction ('falling away') of cells in a growing organism

≈ Latin equivalent ▸**ab-**

---

arch-, archi-
denoting first or primitive
combining form
From Greek ***archē*** = beginning

archenteron	the primitive gut in a developing embryo

---

argent-, argento-
denoting silver
combining form
From Latin ***argentum*** = silver

argentaffin	having an affinity for silver, said of tissues that bind silver salts

≈ Greek equivalent ▸**argyr-, argyro-**

---

argyr-, argyro-
denoting silver
combining form
From Greek ***argyros*** = silver

argyria	a permanent grey discoloration of the skin, caused by excessive ingestion of silver salts
argyrophilic	having an affinity for silver, said of tissues that bind silver salts

≈ Latin equivalent ▸**argent-, argento-**

---

arthr-, arthro-
denoting a joint or joints
combining form
From Greek ***arthron*** = joint

arthritis	inflammation of the joints
arthrodesis	the immobilizing of a joint by the surgical fusion of the bones
arthropathy	a disease of the joints

articular

relating to the joints

adjective

From Latin ***articularis*** = relating to the joints, from ***articulus*** = a small joint, from ***artus*** = a joint

| **articular** rheumatism | rheumatism in the joints |

articulate

having joints

adjective

From Latin ***articulatus*** = divided into joints, from ***articulare*** = to divide into joints

-asthenia

denoting weakness or loss of strength

combining form

From Greek ***astheneia*** = weakness

| my**asthenia** | weakness of the muscles |

◆ Related words **-asthenic** *adj* ▸relating to weakness or loss of strength

asystole

the inability of the heart to pump out blood

noun

From Greek ***a-*** = not and ***systolē*** = contraction, from ***systellein*** = to draw together, to contract, from ***syn*** = together and ***stellein*** = to prepare, to send

◆ Related words **asystolic** *adj* ▸relating to the inability of the heart to pump out blood

-ate

denoting the possession of a particular characteristic

combining form

From Latin ***-atus*** = the past participle ending of verbs ending in ***-are***, corresponding to ***-ed*** in English

| dent**ate** | having teeth, toothed |

atel-, atelo-

denoting the incomplete development of an organ

combining form

From Greek *atelēs* = incomplete, unfinished, imperfect

atelectasis	incomplete inflation of a lung
atelocardia	incomplete development of the heart

ather-, athero-

denoting fatty deposits of a porridge-like consistency

combining form

From Greek *athēra* or *athērē* = gruel, porridge

atherogenic	causing fatty deposits of a porridge-like consistency to develop on the inner surface of arteries
atheroma	a cyst on the inner surface of an artery containing fatty deposits of a porridge-like consistency
atherosclerosis	the thickening of the inner surface of arteries resulting from a build-up of cholesterol and other fatty deposits of a porridge-like consistency

-atric see ▸ -iatric

atrio-

relating to the atria of the heart (▸ **atrium**)

combining form

From Latin *atrium* = entrance hall

atrioventricular	relating to the atria and ventricles of the heart

atrium

either of the two upper cavities of the heart into which blood passes from the veins

noun

From Latin *atrium* = entrance hall

Plural form **atria**

◆ Related words **atrial** *adj* ▸relating to the two upper cavities of the heart

audi-, audio-

denoting the sense of hearing

combining form

From Latin *audire* = to hear

audiology	the study of hearing
audiometer	an instrument for measuring differences in hearing
auditory	relating to the sense, process or organs of hearing

aural

relating to the ear or hearing

adjective

From Latin **auris** = ear

aural anatomy   the anatomy of the ear

≈ Greek equivalent ▸ **otic**

auri-

denoting the ear or hearing

combining form

From Latin **auris** = ear

auriscope   a viewing instrument for examining the ear

≈ Greek equivalent ▸ **ot-, oto-**

auscultate

to listen to internal sounds of the body, such as those of the lungs and heart, as an aid to diagnosis

verb

From Latin **auscultare** = to listen

◆ Related words **auscultation** *n* ▸ the act of listening to the internal sounds of the body; **auscultatory** *adj* ▸ relating to auscultation

aut-, auto-

denoting self

combining form

From Greek **autos** = self

autism   a psychological condition characterized by difficulty in communicating with and relating to others

autoimmune   caused by the reaction of antibodies or immune cells to substances that are naturally present in the body

autointoxication   poisoning by a toxin produced within the body

axillary

relating to, or near, the armpit

adjective

From Latin **axilla** = armpit

axillary artery   the part of the main artery of the arm that is located in the armpit

axillary temperature   a temperature taken by placing a thermometer under the arm

Bb

barba

beard

noun

From Latin ***barba***, genitive ***barbae*** = beard

sycosis **barbae**	inflammation of the hair follicles of the beard
tinea **barbae**	ringworm affecting the beard area of the face

basal

relating to, located at or forming a base; basic

adjective

From Greek ***basis*** = base

basal ganglia	masses of grey matter located at the base of the cerebrum
basal metabolic rate	the rate at which the body uses energy to maintain vital functions while at rest and with an empty stomach

bi-

two, twice

combining form

From Latin ***bis*** = twice

biceps	a muscle with two heads or points of attachment at one end
bicuspid	a tooth with two cusps
bifurcation	division into two branches

! Do not confuse with ▸ **bio-**

≈ Greek equivalent ▸ **di-**

bili-

denoting bile

combining form

From Latin ***bilis*** = bile

biliary	relating to bile, the bile ducts or the gall bladder
bilious	relating to or containing bile

bio-

denoting life or living organisms

combining form

From Greek ***bios*** = life

bioassay the assessment of the strength and effect of a drug or other substance by testing it on a living organism

biochemistry the study of the chemical processes and substances in living organisms

biology the study of living organisms

! Do not confuse with ▸ **bi-**

biotic

relating to living organisms
adjective
From Greek ***biōtikos*** = relating to life

-biotic

denoting living organisms
combining form
From Greek ***biōtikos*** = relating to life

anti**biotic** a substance that can inhibit the growth of, or destroy, micro-organisms that cause infectious diseases

-blast

denoting an immature or embryonic cell or layer of cells
combining form
From Greek ***blastos*** = shoot

epi**blast** the outer germinal layer of an embryo

erythro**blast** a cell in bone marrow that develops into a red blood cell

osteo**blast** a bone-forming cell

blast-, blasto-

denoting embryonic development
combining form
From Greek ***blastos*** = shoot

blastocyst a mammalian embryo at an early stage of development, consisting of a single layer of cells (the *trophectoderm*) surrounding a fluid-filled cavity (*blastocoele*) that contains the inner cell mass

blastomere a cell produced by cleavage of a fertilized ovum in the earliest stages of embryonic development

blastula a clump of cells produced by cleavage divisions of a fertilized egg

blenno-
denoting mucus
combining form
From Greek **blennos** = slime
    blennorrhoea   discharge of mucus

blephar-, blepharo-
denoting the eyelid
combining form
From Greek **blepharon** = eyelid
    blepharitis   inflammation of the eyelid
    blepharoplasty   plastic surgery of the eyelids

brachi-, brachio-
denoting the arm
combining form
From Latin **bracchium** or **brachium** = arm
    brachialgia   pain in the arm
    brachiocephalic   relating to the arms and the head

  ! Do not confuse with ▸ **brachy-**

brachial
relating to the arm
adjective
From Latin **bracchialis** or **brachialis** = relating to the arm
    brachial artery   the artery extending along the inside of the upper part of
                         the arm

  ! Do not confuse with ▸ **branchial**

brachio- see ▸ brachi-, brachio-

brachium
an arm, especially an upper arm
noun
From Latin **bracchium** or **brachium** = arm
Plural form **brachia**

brachy-
short
combining form
From Greek **brachys** = short

brachycephalic   having a short, broad head
brachydactyly   abnormal shortness of the fingers and toes

! Do not confuse with ▸ **brachi-, brachio-**
◑ Opposite ▸ **dolicho-**

---

brady-
slow
combining form
From Greek ***bradys*** = slow

bradycardia   slowness of heartbeat
bradykinesia   slowness of movement, especially as a result of
Parkinson's disease

◑ Opposite ▸ **tachy-**

---

branchial
resembling a gill
adjective
From Latin ***branchia***, from Greek ***branchion*** = gill

branchial cleft   a structure resembling the gill slit of a fish, present in
the neck region of an embryo in the early stages of
development

! Do not confuse with ▸ **brachial; bronchial**

---

bronch-, broncho-
denoting the bronchi (▸ **bronchus**)
combining form
From modern Latin ***bronchus***, from Greek ***bronchos*** = windpipe

bronchitis   inflammation of the lining of the bronchial tubes
bronchodilator   a drug that causes the bronchi to expand

---

bronchial
relating to the bronchi (▸ **bronchus**)
adjective
From modern Latin ***bronchus***, from Greek ***bronchos*** = windpipe

bronchial tubes   the tubes forming the network of airways leading to and
occurring in the lungs

! Do not confuse with ▸ **branchial**

---

broncho- see ▸ bronch-, bronchio-

bronchus

a tube leading from the windpipe to the lung that acts as an airway
noun
From modern Latin ***bronchus***, from Greek ***bronchos*** = windpipe
Plural form **bronchi**

buccal

relating to the cheek or the mouth
adjective
From Latin ***bucca*** = cheek

buccal cavity	the part of the mouth containing the teeth and the tongue

bulla

a blister; a rounded bony protrusion
noun
From Latin ***bulla*** = blister, knob
Plural form **bullae**
◆ Related words **bullous** *adj* ▸relating to a blister or to a rounded bony protrusion

Cc

cac-, caco-

denoting bad or wrong
combining form
From Greek ***kakos*** = bad

cachaemia	an abnormal and chronic condition of the blood
cachexia	a condition of severe physical weakness and wasting of the body associated with severe starvation or chronic disease

callus

an area of thickened or hardened skin; a meshwork of bone that forms around a fracture of a bone
From Latin ***callus*** = hard skin
Plural form **calluses**
◆ Related words **callous** *adj* ▸hardened; relating to a callus

calvaria

the upper part of the skull enclosing the brain

noun

From Latin **calvaria** = skull

calyx

a cup-shaped structure, especially in the pelvis of the kidney

noun

From Greek **kalyx** = husk, cup of a flower

Plural form **calyces** (or **calyxes**)

cancellous

denoting bone that has a spongy or porous structure

adjective

From Latin **cancelli** = lattice

canthus

either corner of the eye where the eyelids meet

noun

From Greek **kanthos** = corner of the eye

Plural form **canthi**

capillary

any of the fine, thin-walled blood vessels that form a network connecting arteries with veins

noun

From Latin **capillaris** = relating to the hair, from **capillus** = hair

capita see ▶ caput

capital

relating to the head; relating to the most prominent part of an organ or structure

adjective

From Latin **capitalis** = relating to the head, from **caput** = head

> slipped **capital** femoral epiphysis   a condition in which the end of the thigh bone slips from the ball of the hip joint

-capnia

denoting carbon dioxide

combining form

From Greek **kapnos** = smoke

| hyper**capnia** | an abnormally high level of carbon dioxide in the blood |
| hypo**capnia** | an abnormally low level of carbon dioxide in the blood |

caput

the head; the most prominent part of an organ or structure

noun

From Latin **caput**, genitive **capitis** = head

Plural form **capita**

| **caput** medusae | dilated veins around the umbilicus in cirrhosis of the liver |
| **caput** succedaneum | swelling on the head of a newborn infant |

carcinoma

a cancer arising in epithelial tissue

noun

From Greek **karkinōma** = cancer, from Greek **karkinos** = crab, cancer

Plural form **carcinomata** (or **carcinomas**)

cardi-, cardio-

denoting the heart or, less frequently, the cardia (the junction between stomach and oesophagus)

combining form

From Greek **kardia** = heart; cardia

carditis	inflammation of the heart
cardiology	the study of the structure, functions and diseases of the heart
cardiovascular	relating to the heart and blood vessels

cardiac

relating to the heart or, less frequently, the cardia (the junction between stomach and oesophagus)

adjective

From Greek **kardiakos** = relating to the heart or the cardia

| **cardiac** arrest | the sudden stopping of the heartbeat |
| **cardiac** muscle | specialized muscle, able to contract rhythmically, found only in the walls of the heart |

cardio- see ▸ cardi-, cardio-

-cardium

denoting the heart

combining form

From modern Latin **cardium**, from Greek **kardia** = heart; cardia (the junction between stomach and oesophagus)

    epi**cardium**   the inner surface of the sac around the heart
    peri**cardium**   the sac around the heart

carp-, carpo-
denoting the wrist
combining form
From modern Latin **carpus**, from Greek **karpos** = wrist

    carpectomy   the surgical removal of all or part of the wrist
    carpopedal spasm   involuntary muscular contraction of the muscles of the hands and feet

carpal
relating to the wrist
adjective
a bone of the wrist
noun
From modern Latin **carpalis**, from modern Latin **carpus**, from Greek **karpos** = wrist

    carpal tunnel syndrome   numbness and pain in the fingers, caused by compression of the nerve as it passes through the space between the bones of the wrist and the tendons

carpo- see ▸ carp-, carpo-

carpus
the wrist
noun
From modern Latin **carpus**, from Greek **karpos** = wrist
Plural form **carpi**

-carpus
denoting the wrist
combining form
From modern Latin **carpus**, from Greek **karpos** = wrist

    meta**carpus**   the part of the hand between the wrist and the fingers

cat-, cata-
down
combining form
From Greek **kata** = down

catabolism	the breaking down by the body of complex molecules, such as carbohydrates or proteins, to produce smaller molecules and liberate energy
cataplexy	a condition of immobility induced by extreme emotion, eg shock (literally 'stricken down')
catheter	a flexible tube inserted into a part of the body so that fluid can travel down it

◗ Opposite ▸ **ana-**

caudal

relating to or located at the lower or 'tail' end of the body
adjective
From modern Latin ***caudalis*** = relating to a tail, from Latin ***cauda*** = tail

| **caudal** vertebra | one of the vertebrae in the coccyx |

-cele

denoting a tumour, hernia or swelling
combining form
From Greek ***kēlē*** = tumour, rupture, hernia

hydro**cele**	a swelling containing serous fluid, especially in the scrotum
meningo**cele**	a protrusion of the meninges through the skull or spine
vario**cele**	a swelling of the veins of the testicle

! Do not confuse with ▸ **-coel, -coele**

-centesis

denoting puncturing
combining form
From Greek ***kentēsis*** = pricking
Plural form **-centeses**

amnio**centesis**	the puncturing of the amnion with a hollow needle to take a sample of the fluid surrounding an embryo
para**centesis**	the puncturing of a body cavity, especially with a hollow needle, to withdraw fluid or gas
thoraco**centesis**	the puncturing of the pleural cavity through the chest wall with a hollow needle to withdraw fluid, blood or air

cephal-, cephalo-

denoting the head
combining form
From Greek ***kephalē*** = head

cephalalgia	headache
cephalometry	the measurement of the head using radiography or ultrasound
cephalotomy	the dissection of the head

-cephalic
-headed
combining form
From Greek **kephalikos** = relating to the head, from Greek **kephalē** = head

| micro**cephalic** | abnormally small-headed |

cephalo- see ▸ cephal-, cephalo-

-cephaly
denoting a particular condition in which the head is of a particular type
combining form
From Greek **kephalē** = head

| macro**cephaly** | abnormal largeness of the head |
| steno**cephaly** | abnormal narrowness of the head |

cerebr-, cerebro-
denoting the cerebrum or the brain
combining form
From Latin **cerebrum** = brain

cerebritis	inflammation of the cerebrum
cerebrospinal	relating to the brain and the spinal cord
cerebrovascular	relating to the brain and its blood vessels

cerebra see ▸ cerebrum

cerebral
relating to the cerebrum or the brain
adjective
From Latin **cerebrum** = brain

| **cerebral** cortex | the outer layer of the front part of the brain |
| **cerebral** hemisphere | either of the halves of the front part of the brain |

cerebrum
the front part of the brain
noun
From Latin **cerebrum** = brain
Plural form **cerebra**

cervic-

denoting the neck of the womb or the neck

combining form

From Latin **cervix**, genitive **cervicis** = neck

| **cervic**algia | neck pain |
| **cervic**itis | inflammation of the neck of the womb |

cervix

the neck of the womb or the neck

combining form

From Latin **cervix** = neck

Plural form **cervices**

◆ Related words **cervical** *adj* ▸relating to the neck of the womb or the neck

chalazion

a small cyst or swelling in the eyelid

noun

From Greek **chalaza** = lump

Plural form **chalazia**

cheil-, cheilo-

denoting the lips

combining form

From Greek **cheilos** = lip

| **cheil**itis | inflammation, dryness and cracking of the lips or the corners of the mouth |
| **cheilo**plasty | plastic surgery of the lips |

≈ Latin equivalent ▸**labi-, labio-**

chir-, chiro-, cheir-, cheiro-

denoting the hand

combining form

From Greek **cheir**, genitive **cheiros** = hand

chiragra	gout in the hand
chiralgia	pain in the hand
chiroplasty	plastic surgery of the hand
chiropractic	a method of treating disorders by manipulation, especially of the spinal column

chlor-, chloro-

denoting green; denoting chlorine

combining form

chol-, chole-

From Greek **chlōros** = pale green

chloroform   a colourless volatile liquid that is a compound of carbon, hydrogen and chlorine, formerly used as a general anaesthetic

chloropsia   a disorder of the vision in which everything appears green

chol-, chole-
denoting bile, the bile ducts or gall
combining form
From Greek **cholē** = bile, gall

cholaemia   the presence of bile pigments in the blood

cholagogue   a substance that causes bile to flow from the gall bladder into the duodenum

cholelithiasis   the presence of gallstones in the gall bladder and bile ducts

choledoch-, choledocho-
denoting the common bile duct
combining form
From Greek **cholēdochos** = containing bile

choledochectomy   the surgical removal of part of the common bile duct

choledocho-lithiasis   the presence of gallstones in the common bile duct

choledochotomy   a surgical incision into the common bile duct

chondr-, chondri-, chondro-
denoting cartilage
combining form
From Greek **chondros** = cartilage

a**chondro**plasia   a hereditary disorder in which cartilage fails to convert to bone so that dwarfism results

chondrify   to convert tissue into cartilage, or be converted into cartilage

chondrocranium   the skull of an embryo, composed of cartilage which eventually becomes bone

chord-, chordo-
denoting a cord, tendon or nerve fibre
combining form
From Latin **chorda**, from Greek **chordē** = gut, gut string

chorditis   inflammation of a cord, especially a vocal cord

chordotomy the surgical division of bundles of nerve fibres in the spinal cord to relieve severe or persistent pain

---

chorda

a cord, tendon or nerve fibre

noun

From Latin ***chorda***, from Greek ***chordē*** = gut, gut string

Plural form **chordae**

chordae tendineae stringlike structures that attach the heart valves to the papillary muscles

---

chordo- see ▸ chord-, chordo-

---

chorio-

denoting the outer membrane surrounding the embryo, which develops into the placenta as the embryo grows

combining form

From Greek ***chorion*** = membrane surrounding the embryo

choriocarcinoma a malignant tumour originating in the outer membrane surrounding the embryo

---

chorion

the outer membrane surrounding the embryo, which develops into the placenta as the embryo grows

noun

From Greek ***chorion*** = membrane surrounding the embryo

Plural form **choria**

◆ Related words **chorionic** or **chorial** *adj* ▸ relating to the the chorion

---

choroid

the vascular membrane of the eyeball, between the retina and the sclera

noun

relating to or resembling the membrane surrounding the embryo (the chorion)

adjective

From Greek ***choroeidēs*** = resembling the membrane surrounding the embryo

choroid plexus a vascular membrane projecting into the ventricles of the brain and secreting cerebrospinal fluid

---

chrom-, chromo-

denoting colour

combining form

From Greek ***chrōma*** = colour

| a**chrom**ia | loss of pigmentation |
| **chromo**some | any of the deeply staining rod-like structures seen in the nucleus at cell division |

---

chron-, chrono-
denoting time
combining form
From Greek ***chronos*** = time

| **chron**axie | a time constant in the excitation of a nerve or muscle which equals the smallest time required to produce a response when the stimulus is double the minimum intensity required to produce a basic response |
| **chrono**biology | the study of biological rhythms |

---

chrys-, chryso-
denoting gold
combining form
From Greek ***chrysos*** = gold

| **chryso**therapy | the treatment of disease using gold salts |

---

cicatrix or cicatrice
a scar
noun
From Latin ***cicatrix***, genitive ***cicatricis*** = scar
Plural form **cicatrices** (or **cicatrixes**)
◆ Related words **cicatricial** *adj* ▸relating to scarring

-cidal
denoting killing
combining form
From Latin ***caedere*** = to kill

| bacteri**cidal** | killing bacteria |

-cide
denoting killing, killer
combining form
From Latin ***caedere*** = to kill

| germi**cide** | a substance that kills germs |
| sui**cide** | the killing of oneself |

ciliary

relating to the hair-like structures found on the surface of an epithelial cell;
relating to the part of the eye connecting the iris to the vascular membrane
of the eyeball

adjective

From Latin *cilium* = eyelid

ciliary body	the part of the eye connecting the iris to the vascular membrane of the eyeball
ciliary muscle	the muscle in the ciliary body that contracts to alter the shape of the lens and change its focus

cilium

an eyelash; one of the hair-like structures found on the surface of an
epithelial cell

noun

From Latin *cilium* = eyelid

Plural form **cilia**

circum-

around

combining form

From Latin *circum* = around

circumanal	around the anus
circumcision	the cutting off of the foreskin or clitoris
circumoral	around the mouth

≈ Greek equivalent ▸**peri-**

-clast

denoting something that breaks or absorbs something else

combining form

From Greek *klastēs* = breaker, from *klaein* = to break

odonto**clast**	a cell that absorbs the roots of milk teeth
osteo**clast**	a cell that absorbs bone (*physiol*); a surgical instrument for fracturing bone (*surg*)

claudication

lameness

noun

From Latin *claudicatio* = a limping, from Latin *claudus* = lame

intermittent **claudication**	a cramp-like pain in one or both legs that develops on walking, caused by eg atherosclerosis

cleid-, cleido-

denoting the collarbone

combining form

From Greek *kleis*, genitive *kleidos* = bar, bolt, hook, key, collarbone

cleidocranial	relating to the collarbone and cranium
cleidotomy	the cutting of the collarbones of a fetus to make delivery easier

clonus

a type of spasm in which a muscle undergoes a series of rapid contractions and relaxations

noun

From modern Latin, from Greek *klonos* = turmoil

◆ Related words **clonic** *adj* ▸relating to a type of spasm in which a muscle undergoes a series of rapid contractions and relaxations

-cnemial

denoting the shin or tibia

combining form

From Greek *knēmē* = lower leg, tibia

gastro**cnemial**	relating to the main muscle of the calf of the leg

-cnemius

denoting the shin or tibia

combining form

From Greek *knēmē* = lower leg, tibia

Plural form **-cnemii**

gastro**cnemius**	the main muscle of the calf of the leg

coccyges see ▸ coccyx

co-, com-, con-

together, with, similar

combining form

From Latin *cum* = with

coarctation	the narrowing or drawing together of the aorta
coenzyme	a non-protein organic molecule that bonds with a specific enzyme only while the biochemical reaction is being catalysed, being essential to, but unaffected by, the reaction
commensal	an organism living in partnership or association with another of a different species without affecting or benefiting it

congenital   dating from birth, but not necessarily hereditary

conjoined twins   a set of twins who are physically joined together

≈ Greek equivalent ▸ **sy-, syl-, sym-, syn-, sys-**

---

coccyg-, coccygo-
relating to the coccyx
combining form
From Greek ***kokkyx***, genitive ***kokkygos*** = cuckoo, coccyx

coccygectomy   the surgical removal of the coccyx

coccygodynia   pain in the coccyx

coccygotomy   the surgical cutting of the coccyx

---

coccyx
the terminal triangular bone of the vertebral column, consisting of four tiny bones fused together and shaped like a cuckoo's beak
noun
From Greek ***kokkyx***, genitive ***kokkygos*** = cuckoo, coccyx
Plural form **coccyges** (or **coccyxes**)
◆ Related words **coccygeal** *adj* ▸ relating to the coccyx

---

coel-, coelo-
denoting a cavity in the body
combining form
From Greek ***koilos*** = hollow

coeloscope   a viewing instrument for examining the interior of a body cavity

! Do not confuse with ▸ **coeli-, coelio-**

-coel, -coele
denoting a cavity in the body
combining form
From Greek ***koilos*** = hollow

blasto**coele**   the cavity inside a mammalian embryo at an early stage of development

! Do not confuse with ▸ **-cele**

---

coeli-, coelio-
denoting the abdomen
combining form
From Greek ***koilia*** = abdomen

| **coeli**ectasia | abnormal swelling of the abdomen |
| **coelio**scopy | an examination of interior of the abdomen with a viewing instrument |

! Do not confuse with ▸ **coel-, coelo-**

coeliac

relating to the abdomen (*anat*); relating to coeliac disease (*pathol*)
adjective
someone who has coeliac disease
noun
From Latin ***coeliacus***, from Greek ***koiliakos***, from Greek ***koilia*** = abdomen

| **coeliac** disease | a condition of the intestines in which a sensitivity to gluten prevents the proper absorption of nutrients |
| **coeliac** trunk | a branch of the abdominal artery that itself divides into branches supplying blood to the stomach, liver and spleen |

coelio- see ▸ coeli-, coelio-

col-, coli-, colo-

denoting the colon
combining form
From Greek ***kōlon*** = limb, member

colectomy	the surgical removal of all or part of the colon
coliform bacteria	rod-shaped bacteria found in the colon
colitis	inflammation of the colon
colorectal	relating to the colon and the rectum

columella

any of various column-like anatomical structures, such as the central column of the cochlea or the fleshy lower part of the nasal septum
noun
From Latin ***columella*** = little column, from ***columna*** = column
Plural form **columellae** (or **columellas**)

colp-, colpo-

denoting the vagina
combining form
From Greek ***kolpos*** = bosom, lap, womb, vagina

colpitis	inflammation of the vagina
colposcope	a viewing instrument for examining the vagina and cervix
colpoptosis	a prolapse of the vagina

com- see ▸ **co-, com-, con-**

con- see ▸ **co-, com-, con-**

condyle
a rounded protuberance at the end of a bone for articulation with another bone, such as the ball in a ball-and-socket joint
noun
From Latin ***condylus***, from Greek ***kondylos*** = knuckle
◆ Related words **condylar** *adj* ▸relating to a condyle
condyloid *adj* ▸resembling a condyle

condyl-, condylo-
denoting a rounded protuberance, especially one at the end of a bone for articulation with another bone, such as the ball in a ball-and-socket joint
combining form
From Latin ***condylus***, from Greek ***kondylos*** = knuckle

condyloma	a rounded warty growth on the skin or mucous membrane around the genitals or anus

contra-
against, opposite, contrary
combining form
From Latin contra = against

contraceptive	a drug, device or other means of preventing unwanted pregnancy
contraindication	any factor in a patient's condition which indicates that a treatment would involve a greater than normal degree of risk and is therefore unwise to pursue
contralateral	located on or affecting the opposite side of the body

≈ Greek equivalent ▸ **anti-**

copr-, copro-
denoting faeces
combining form
From Greek ***kopros*** = excrement, dung

copremesis	the vomiting of faeces
coprolalia	obsessive or repetitive use of obscene language, eg as a characteristic of Tourette's syndrome
coprophilia	an abnormal interest in faeces or defecation

≈ Latin equivalent ▸ **faeco-; sterc-, sterco-, stercor-, stercori-**

cor

the heart

noun

From Latin **cor**, genitive **cordis** = heart

Plural form **corda**

cor pulmonale	pulmonary heart disease
cor triloculare	a congenital condition in which the heart has only three chambers instead of four

-cordial

relating to the heart

combining form

From Latin **cor**, genitive **cordis** = heart

pre**cordial**	in front of the heart

corium

the true skin, below the outer layer

noun

From Latin **corium** = skin, hide, leather

◆ Related words **corious** *adj* ▸relating to the corium

corona

a crown or a structure resembling a crown

noun

From Latin **corona** = wreath, crown

Plural form **coronae** or **coronas**

corona capitis	the crown of the head

coronal

relating to the crown of the head; relating to the coronal plane

adjective

From Latin **coronalis** = relating to a crown, from Latin **corona** = wreath, crown

coronal plane	an imaginary plane down the middle of the body splitting it into front and back parts
coronal suture	the serrated line across the skull separating the frontal bone from the parietal bones

coronary

relating to the region around an organ, especially the heart

adjective

From Latin **coronarius** = relating to a wreath or crown, from Latin **corona** = wreath, crown

| **coronary** artery | one of the branching arteries supplying blood to the heart wall from the aorta |
| **coronary** thrombosis | a stoppage in a branch of a coronary artery by a clot of blood, which causes part of the heart muscle to die |

◀▶ Related words **coronary** *noun* ▸a coronary thrombosis

---

corpus

any mass of body tissue that may be distinguished from its surroundings
noun
From Latin *corpus*, genitive *corporis* = body
Plural form **corpora**

| **corpus** callosum | a broad band of nerve fibre between the two cerebral hemispheres |
| **corpus** luteum | a mass of yellow glandular tissue that develops in a Graafian follicle after the eruption of an ovum and secretes progesterone to prepare the uterus for implantation |

◀▶ Related words **corporeal** *adj* ▸relating to the body

---

cortex

the outer layer of some organs, especially the brain
noun
From Latin *cortex*, genitive *corticis* = bark, covering
Plural form **cortices**

adrenal **cortex**	the outer part of an adrenal gland
cerebral **cortex**	the outer layer of the front part of the brain
renal **cortex**	the outer layer of a kidney

◀▶ Related words **cortical** *adj* ▸relating to a cortex

---

cortico-

denoting the outer layer of some organs
combining form
From Latin *cortex*, genitive *corticis* = bark, covering

| **cortico**steroid | any steroid hormone, eg cortisone, synthesized by the adrenal cortex; a group of drugs derived from or similar to naturally produced corticosteroid hormones |
| **cortico**sterone | a steroid hormone secreted by the adrenal cortex |

---

cost-, costo-

denoting a rib or the ribs
combining form
From Latin *costa* = rib

costectomy	the surgical removal of a rib
costotomy	the surgical cutting of a rib

costal

relating to a rib or the ribs

adjective

From modern Latin ***costalis***, from Latin ***costa*** = rib

costal cartilage	a cartilage connecting a rib to the breastbone

-costal

denoting a rib or the ribs

combining form

From modern Latin ***costalis***, from Latin ***costa*** = rib

inter**costal**	between the ribs

costo- see ▸ cost-, costo-

cox-, coxo-

denoting a hip bone or hip joint

combining form

From Latin ***coxa*** = hip, hip bone

coxalgia	pain in the hip joint; disease of the hip joint
coxodynia	pain in the hip joint
coxofemoral	relating to the hip bone and the femur

coxa

a hip bone or hip joint

noun

From Latin ***coxa*** = hip, hip bone

Plural form **coxae**

◆▸ Related words **coxal** *adj* ▸relating to a hip bone or hip joint

coxo- see ▸ cox-, coxo-

crani-, cranio-

denoting the skull or cranium

combining form

From medieval Latin, from Greek ***kranion*** = skull

craniectomy	the surgical removal of a piece of the skull
craniosacral therapy	an alternative therapy involving gentle manipulation of the bones and membranes of the skull, in order to treat a wide range of physical and psychological disorders

cranial

relating to the skull or cranium

adjective

From medieval Latin, from Greek **kranion** = skull

cranial nerve   any of the twelve pairs of nerves originating in the brain

---

cranio- see ▸ crani-, cranio-

---

crepitus

crackling sounds produced by the friction between the surfaces of joints or broken bones, or by the lungs in pneumonia

noun

From Latin **crepitus** = rattling, creaking

-crine

denoting secretion

combining form

From Greek **krinein** = to separate

endo**crine** gland   a gland that produces and secretes hormones directly into the bloodstream

exo**crine** gland   a gland that secretes its products through a duct that opens onto an epithelial surface

---

crista

a crest or ridge (*anat*); a fold of the inner membrane of a mitochondrion (*biol*)

noun

From Latin **crista** = tuft, cockscomb, crest

Plural form **cristae**

---

cruciate

cross-shaped or arranged like a cross

adjective

From modern Latin **cruciatus**, from Latin **crux**, genitive **crucis** = cross

cruciate ligament   one of a pair of ligaments that cross each other in the knee, connecting the femur and the tibia

---

crus

a leg, especially a lower leg; an elongated structure in the body, especially one of a pair

noun

From Latin **crus**, genitive **cruris** = leg

Plural form **crura**

crus cerebri   one of a pair of symmetrical nerve tracts in the midbrain

◆ Related words **crural** *adj* ▸relating to a leg or an elongated structure in the body

---

cry-, cryo-
denoting low temperature or freezing
combining form
From Greek **kryos** = icy cold, frost

cryaesthesia   hypersensitivity to low temperature; a cold sensation

cryosurgery   surgery using instruments at very low temperatures to cut and destroy tissue

cryotherapy   medical treatment using extreme cold

---

crypt-, crypto-
denoting hidden
combining form
From Greek **kryptos** = hidden, secret

cryptogenic disease   a disease with an unknown or obscure cause

cryptorchidism   a condition in which one or both testes fail to descend into the scrotum

---

cubital
relating to the elbow or forearm
adjective
From Latin **cubitalis** = relating to the elbow, from Latin **cubitum** = elbow

cubital fossa   the triangular depression in the arm at the front of the elbow

---

cutaneous
relating to the skin
adjective
From modern Latin **cutaneus**, from Latin **cutis** = skin

-cutaneous
denoting the skin
combining form
From modern Latin **cutaneus**, from Latin **cutis** = skin

sub**cutaneous**   beneath or just under the skin

---

cutis
the true skin, below the outer layer
noun

From Latin **cutis** = skin

cyan-, cyano-
denoting blue
combining form
From Greek **kyanos** = dark blue

cyanopathy	a disease characterized by bluish discoloration of the skin resulting from lack of oxygen in the blood
cyanosis	bluish discoloration of the skin resulting from lack of oxygen in the blood

cycl-, cyclo-
denoting a circle or cycle; denoting the ciliary body of the eye
combining form
From Greek **kyklos** = circle, cycle

cyclectomy	the surgical removal of the ciliary body of the eye
cyclophoria	a type of squint in which the eye rotates clockwise or anticlockwise
cyclothymia	a psychiatric disorder characterized by periodic mood swings from elation to misery

cyesis
pregnancy
noun
From Greek **kyēsis** = conception, pregnancy
Plural form **cyeses**

-cyesis
denoting pregnancy
combining form
From Greek **kyēsis** = conception, pregnancy

pseudo**cyesis**	phantom pregnancy

Plural form **-cyeses**

cyst
a sac or vesicle in the body (*anat*); a sac that forms in the body containing diseased fluid or semisolid matter (*pathol*)
adjective
From late Latin **cystis**, from Greek **kystis** = bladder

dermoid **cyst**	a cyst of similar cell structure to that of skin, usually congenital or occurring in the ovary
hydatid **cyst**	a water cyst or vesicle in the body, especially one containing a tapeworm larva

cyst-, cysto-

denoting the bladder; denoting a cyst

combining form

From late Latin **cystis**, from Greek **kystis** = bladder

cystectomy	the surgical removal of the urinary bladder; the surgical removal of an abnormal cyst
cystitis	inflammation of the inner lining of the urinary bladder
cystoscope	an instrument inserted up the urethra for examination of the urinary bladder

≈ Latin equivalent ▸ **vesic-, vesico-**

cyt-, cyto-

denoting a cell

combining form

From Greek **kytos** = hollow, vessel, container

cytology	the study of the structure and function of individual cells
cytoplasm	the protoplasm of a cell surrounding the nucleus

-cyte

denoting a cell

combining form

From Greek **kytos** = hollow, vessel, container

leuco**cyte**	a white blood cell
osteo**cyte**	a bone cell
phago**cyte**	a white blood cell that engulfs bacteria and other harmful particles

cyto- see ▸ **cyt-, cyto-**

Dd

dacry-, dacryo-

denoting tears

combining form

From Greek **dakryon** = tear

dacryagogue	a substance that causes the lachrymal glands to secrete tears
dacryoadenitis	inflammation of the lachrymal gland

dactyl-, dactylo-

denoting a finger or toe

combining form

From Greek **daktylos** = finger, toe

dactylitis	inflammation of a finger or toe
dactylomegaly	a condition in which someone has abnormally large fingers and toes

-dactyly

denoting an abnormal congenital condition of the fingers and toes

combining form

From Greek **daktylos** = finger, toe

brachy**dactyly**	abnormal shortness of the fingers and toes
hypo**dactyly**	a congenital condition in which someone has fewer fingers or toes than normal
poly**dactyly**	a congenital condition in which someone has more than the normal number of fingers or toes
syn**dactyly**	a congenital condition in which the fingers or toes are fused together

de-

denoting removal, separation, loss, reversal

combining form

From Latin **de** = from, away from

decalcification	the loss or removal of calcium from bones or teeth
decongestant	a substance that relieves nasal congestion
defibrillation	the application of an electric current to the heart to restore the normal rhythm after fibrillation has occurred

deci-

denoting one tenth

combining form

From Latin **decimus** = tenth

decibel	a unit for measuring the intensity of sound, equivalent to one tenth of a bel
decilitre	one tenth of a litre

decidua

a membrane that lines the uterus and is discharged after childbirth

noun

From Latin **deciduus** = falling down, falling off

Plural form **deciduae** (or **deciduas**)

deciduous

liable to be shed at a certain period

adjective

From Latin ***deciduus*** = falling down, falling off

deciduous teeth   milk teeth

---

deltoid

the large triangular muscle of the shoulder

noun

From Greek ***deltoeidēs*** = delta-shaped, triangular, from ***delta*** = delta or Δ, the fourth letter of the Greek alphabet

---

dem-, demo-

denoting people or population

combining form

From Greek ***dēmos*** = people

demography   the study of population, especially with reference to size, density and distribution

---

demi-

denoting half or half-sized

combining form

From medieval Latin ***dimedius***, from Latin ***dimidius*** = half

demifacet   one of a pair of small flat areas formed when the head of a bone articulates with the bases of a pair of adjacent vertebrae

≈ Greek equivalent ▸**hemi-**

-demic

denoting people

combining form

From Greek ***dēmos*** = people

epi**demic**   a disease that attacks great numbers of people in one place at one time, and itself travels from place to place

pan**demic**   a disease that attacks great numbers of people in many different countries

---

demo- see ▸**dem-, demo-**

---

dendrite

a branching projection of a nerve cell

noun

From Greek ***dendritēs*** = relating to a tree, from ***dendron*** = tree

40

dendritic

branching; relating to a a branching projection of a nerve cell

adjective

From Greek **dendritēs** = relating to a tree, from **dendron** = tree

dendritic ulcer — an ulcer with a branching structure affecting the surface of the cornea and caused by the herpes simplex virus

dendritic cell — a cell with branching projections

dent-, denti-, dento-

denoting a tooth or teeth

combining form

From Latin **dens**, genitive **dentis** = tooth

dentilabial — relating to the teeth and the lips

dentition — the cutting or growing of teeth; the shape, number, and typical arrangement of the teeth

dentoalveolar — relating to a tooth and its socket

≈ Greek equivalent ▸ **odont-, odonto-**

dental

relating to the teeth or dentistry

adjective

From medieval Latin **dentalis**, from Latin **dens**, genitive **dentis** = tooth

dental caries — tooth decay

inferior **dental** nerve — the nerve supplying the lower set of teeth

superior **dental** nerve — the nerve supplying the upper set of teeth

dentate

toothed

adjective

From Latin **dentatus** = toothed, having teeth

dentate gyrus — a fold on the surface of the hippocampus

denti-, dento- see ▸ dent-

derm, derma, dermis

the true skin, below the outer layer

noun

From Greek **derma**, genitive **dermatos** = skin

dermat-, dermato-

dermat-, dermato-
denoting the skin
combining form
From Greek **derma**, genitive **dermatos** = skin

dermatitis	inflammation of the skin
dermatophyte	a parasitic fungus of the skin
dermatosis	a disease of the skin, especially one without inflammation

dermis see ▸ **derm, derma, dermis**

-desis
denoting binding together
combining form
From Greek **desis** = binding together

arthro**desis**	the immobilizing of a joint in the body by the surgical fusion of the bones

deut-, deuter-, deutero-, deuto-
denoting second or secondary
combining form
From Greek **deuteros** = second

deuteranopia	a type of colour blindness in which red and green are confused, blue and yellow only being distinguished
deutoplasm	the food material, such as yolk or fat, within an egg or cell

dextr-, dextro-
denoting on or to the right
combining form
From Latin **dexter**, genitive **dextri** = on or to the right

dextrocardia	a condition in which the heart lies in the right side of the chest, not the left
dextrose	glucose

◑ Opposite ▸ **laev-, laevo-, lev-, levo-; sinistr-, sinistro-**

di-
twice, double, two
combining form
From Greek **dis** = twice, doubly

dichromatic	able to see only two of the three primary colours
dicrotism	a condition in which the pulse has two beats per beat of the heart

! Do not confuse with ▸ **di-, dia-**

≈ Latin equivalent ▸ **bi-**

---

di-, dia-
through, throughout, apart
combining form
From Greek **dia** = through, across

diakinesis	the final stage of the first phase of meiosis, during which pairs of homologous chromosomes almost completely separate
dialysis	the removal of impurities from the blood by a kidney machine
diarrhoea	a condition in which liquid faeces are persistently discharged from the bowels
diuretic	a medicine or other substance that increases the flow of urine

! Do not confuse with ▸ **di-**
≈ Latin equivalent ▸ **per-**

---

diastole
the dilatation of the heart, atria and arteries
noun
From Greek **diastolē** = dilatation, from **diastellein** = to dilate, from **dia** = apart and **stellein** = to prepare, to send
◆ Related words **diastolic** *adj* ▸ relating to the dilatation of the heart, atria and arteries

---

digital
relating to the fingers
adjective
From Latin **digitus** = finger, toe

digital rectal exam	an examination of the rectum using a finger or fingers

---

dipl-, diplo-
denoting double; denoting possessing two sets of chromosomes, one set coming from each parent
combining form
From Greek **diplous** = double

diplopia	double vision
diplotene	the fourth stage of the first phase of meiosis, in which the chromosomes clearly double

diploid

having two sets of chromosomes, one set coming from each parent
adjective
From Greek **diplous** = double and **-oeidēs** = resembling, having the form of, from **eidos** = form, shape

-dipsia

denoting thirst
combining form
From Greek **dipsa** = thirst

   poly**dipsia**   excessive thirst

dipso-

denoting thirst
combining form
From Greek **dipsa** = thirst

   dipsomania   an intermittent pathological craving for alcohol

dis-

denoting apart, reversal
combining form
From Latin **dis** = apart

   disarticulation   the separation of bones at a joint
   disinfection   the process of destroying bacteria that cause disease
   dislocation   the displacement of a bone from its joint
   dissection   the act of cutting in pieces a body in order to ascertain the structure of its parts

! Do not confuse with ▸ **dys-**

distal

farthest from the point of attachment (*anat*); farthest from the centre (*dent*)
adjective
From Latin **distare** = to be distant
◑ Opposite ▸ **proximal**

dolicho-

denoting long
combining form
From Greek **dolichos** = long

   dolichocephalic   having a long, narrow head

◑ Opposite ▸ **brachy-**

dolori-

denoting pain

combining form

From Latin *dolor*, genitive *doloris* = pain

dolorimetry   the measurement of sensitivity to pain

-dontia see ▸ -odontia

---

dors-, dorsi-, dorso-

denoting the back of the body; denoting backwards

combining form

From Latin *dorsum* = back

dorsalgia   back pain

dorsiflexion   the bending back of the hand, foot, fingers or toes

dorsoventral   relating to the back and front of the body

---

dorsal

relating to the back of the body or an organ

adjective

From Latin *dorsum* = back

dorsal vertebra   a vertebra of the spine

◗ Opposite ▸ **ventral**

---

dorsi-, dorso- see ▸ dors-, dorsi-, dorso-

-duct

denoting a tube

combining form

From Latin *ductus* = leading, conducting, from *ducere* = to lead, to conduct, to draw

ovi**duct**   the tube that conveys an egg from the ovary to the uterus

---

-duction

denoting leading, conducting

combining form

From Latin *ductio* = leading, from *ducere* = to lead, to conduct, to draw

trans**duction**   the transfer of genetic material from one bacterial cell to another by bacteriophage

-ductor

denoting something that leads or conducts something else in a particular direction

combining form

From Latin ***ductor*** = leader, from ***ducere*** = to lead, to conduct, to draw

ad**ductor**	a muscle which, when it contracts, moves a body part towards the midline of the body

duo-

denoting two

combining form

From Latin ***duo*** = two

duopoly	a situation in which two companies etc are the only suppliers in a particular market

duoden-, duodeno-

denoting the first portion of the small intestine (so called because it is about twelve fingers'-breadth in length)

combining form

From Latin ***duodeni*** = twelve each

duodenectomy	the surgical removal of the first portion of the small intestine
duodenitis	inflammation of the first portion of the small intestine
duodenoscope	a viewing instrument for examining the interior of the first portion of the small intestine

duodenal

relating to the first portion of the small intestine (so called because it is about twelve fingers'-breadth in length)

adjective

From Latin ***duodeni*** = twelve each

duodenal ulcer	an ulcer in the first portion of the small intestine

duodenum

the first portion of the small intestine (so called because it is about twelve fingers'-breadth in length)

noun

From Latin ***duodeni*** = twelve each

Plural form **duodena**

dura (mater)

the exterior membrane of the brain and spinal column

noun

From Latin **durus** = hard and **mater** = mother
◆ Related words **dural** *adj* ▸relating to the exterior membrane of the brain and spinal column

---

-dynia see ▸ **-odynia**

---

dys-
denoting bad, difficult, painful, impaired or abnormal
combining form
From Greek **dys-** = hard, bad, unlucky

dysfunction	impairment or abnormality of the functioning of an organ
dysmenorrhoea	difficult or painful menstruation
dysplasia	abnormal development or growth of a cell, tissue, organ, etc
dystrophy	any of several disorders in which there is wasting of muscle tissue etc

! Do not confuse with ▸ **dis-**
◑ Opposite ▸ **eu-**

Ee

---

e-, ex-
out, outside
combining form
From Latin **e** or **ex** = out of, from

evaginate	to turn an organ inside out
excision	the surgical cutting out of tissue, an organ or a tumour
excretion	the discharge of waste products from the bowels, bladder, sweat glands, etc
exhalation	the act of breathing out used air

! Do not confuse with ▸ **exo-**
≈ Greek equivalent ▸ **ec-, ex-**

---

ec-, ex-
out
combining form
From Greek **ek** or **ex** = out of, from

ecbolic	a drug that induces contractions of the uterus leading to childbirth or abortion

| **ex**ophthalmos | a condition in which the eyeballs protrude from their sockets |
| **ex**ostosis | a benign outgrowth of cartilage from a bone |

! Do not confuse with ▸ **exo-**
≈ Latin equivalent ▸ **e-, ex-**

---

ectasis

the abnormal dilation of a duct, tube or hollow organ
noun
From Greek ***ektasis*** = stretching out, extension
Plural form **ectases**

-ectasis

denoting the dilation of a duct, tube or hollow organ
combining form
From Greek ***ektasis*** = stretching out, extension
Plural form **-ectases**

atel**ectasis**	incomplete inflation of a lung
bronchi**ectasis**	a chronic disease caused by dilated bronchi
telangi**ectasis**	dilatation of the small arteries or capillaries

---

ecto-

outside, outer, external
combining form
From Greek ***ektos*** = outside

| **ecto**derm | the outer layer of cells of an embryo in the early stages of development, or the tissues directly derived from this layer |
| **ecto**genesis | the development of an embryo outside the body in an artificial environment |

! Do not confuse with ▸ **ectro-; exo-**
◑ Opposite ▸ **end-, endo-; ent-, ento-**

-ectomy

denoting the surgical removal of a part of the body
combining form
From Greek ***ektomē*** = cutting out, excision

| append**ectomy** | the surgical removal of the appendix |
| mast**ectomy** | the surgical removal of a breast |

ectopia

the abnormal displacement of an organ or part

noun

From Greek ***ektopos*** = away from a place, from ***ek*** = out of, from and
topos = place

ectopic

in an abnormal position

adjective

From Greek ***ektopos*** = away from a place, from ***ek*** = out of, from and ***topos*** =
place

    ectopic pregnancy the development of a fetus outside the uterus, especially
                    in a Fallopian tube

ectro-

denoting the congenital absence of an organ or body part

combining form

From Greek ***ektrōma*** = abortion

    ectrodactyly   the congenital absence of all or part of one or more
                          fingers or toes

    ectromelia   the congenital absence of all or part of one or more limbs

   ! Do not confuse with ▸**ecto-**

efferent

conveying away from a body part or organ

adjective

From Latin ***efferens***, genitive ***efferentis*** = carrying away, from ***ex*** = from and
ferre = to carry

    efferent nerve   a nerve that conveys impulses from the brain or spinal
                      cord

   ◑ Opposite ▸**afferent**

em- see ▸en-, em-

embryo

an unborn vertebrate in the earliest stages of development, especially a
developing human in the first eight weeks after conception

noun

From late Latin, from Greek ***embryon*** = embryo, foetus, from ***en*** = in and
bryein = to swell

   ◖ Related words **embryonic** *adj* ▸relating to an embryo

embryo-

denoting an unborn vertebrate in the earliest stages of development, especially a developing human in the first eight weeks after conception

combining form

From late Latin, from Greek **embryon** = embryo, foetus, from **en** = in and **bryein** = to swell

embryogenesis	the formation and development of an embryo
embryology	the study of the formation and development of embryos

emesis

vomiting

noun

From Greek **emesis** = vomiting

emetic

causing vomiting

adjective

a medicine that causes vomiting

noun

From Greek **emetikos** = causing vomiting

emeto-

denoting vomiting

combining form

From Greek **emetos** = vomiting

emetophobia	a pathological fear of vomiting

en-, em-

denoting in, into

combining form

From Greek **en** = in, into

embolus	a blockage in a blood vessel consisting of a clot, air bubble or fatty deposit
emphysema	an unnatural distension of the lungs, which causes breathing difficulties
enema	a fluid injected into the rectum, or the process of injecting such a fluid
enophthalmos	a condition in which the eyeballs are located abnormally deeply in their sockets

encephal-, encephalo-

denoting the brain

combining form

From Greek **enkephalos** = brain, from **en** = in and **kephalē** = head

encephalitis	inflammation of the brain
encephalography	radiography of the brain
encephalomyelitis	inflammation of the brain and spinal cord
encephalopathy	a degenerative brain disease

end-, endo-
within, inside
combining form
From Greek **endon** = within

endarterectomy	the surgical removal of material obstructing blood flow in an artery
endometrium	the mucous membrane lining the cavity of the uterus
endoscope	a viewing instrument for examining the cavities of internal organs
endothelium	the layer of cell tissue on the internal surfaces of blood vessels, lymphatics, etc

! Do not confuse with ▸ **ent-, ento-**
≈ Latin equivalent ▸ **intra-**
◑ Opposite ▸ **ecto-**

ent-, ento-
within, inside
combining form
From Greek **entos** = within, inside

entoptic	occurring within the eyeball, or relating to the visibility to the eye of objects within itself
entotic	relating to the interior of the ear
entozoon	an animal that lives as a parasite within the body of its host

! Do not confuse with ▸ **end-, endo-**
≈ Latin equivalent ▸ **intra-**
◑ Opposite ▸ **ecto-**

enter-, entero-
denoting the intestine
combining form
From Greek **enteron** = intestine

enterectomy	the surgical removal of part of the intestine
enterocentesis	the puncturing of the intestine with a hollow needle to withdraw fluid or gas or to insert a catheter

| **entero**pathy | an intestinal disorder |
| **entero**virus | any of several viruses occurring in and infecting the intestine |

ento- see ▸ ent-, ento-

ep-, epi-
denoting on, upon, over, above, near, after, in addition
combining form
From Greek *epi* = on, upon, over, above, near, after, in addition to

epiblast	the outer germinal layer of an embryo
epidermis	the outer layer of the skin that forms a protective covering over the true skin or dermis
epiglottis	a flap of cartilage over the glottis
epiphenomenon	a secondary symptom of a disease

episio-
denoting the vulva
combining form
From Greek *epision* = pubic region

| **episio**stenosis | a narrowing of the opening of the vulva |
| **episio**tomy | an incision made in the perineum to facilitate the delivery of a baby |

equi-
denoting equal
combining form
From Latin *aequus* = equal

| **equi**distant | equally distant |

erg-, ergo-
denoting work
combining form
From Greek *ergon* – work

| **ergo**meter | an instrument for measuring the work done by the muscles during physical avticity |

-ergic
denoting action, activity, production
combining form
From Greek *ergon* = work

| adren**ergic** | releasing or activated by adrenaline or a substance resembling adrenaline |

| cholin**ergic** | releasing or activated by acetylcholine |

ergo- see ▸**erg-, ergo-**

erot-, eroto-
    denoting sexual desire
    combining form
    From Greek *erōs*, genitive *erōtos* = (sexual) love

| **eroto**mania | an obsessive condition in which someone believes that another person is in love with them |
| **eroto**phobia | a fear of or aversion to any form of sexual involvement |

eryth-, erythr-, erythro-
    denoting red; denoting red blood cells
    combining form
    From Greek *erythros* = red

erythema	redness of the skin
erythroblast	a cell in bone marrow that develops into a red blood cell
erythrocyte	a red blood cell
erythropoiesis	the formation of red blood cells

eu-
    denoting well, good, easy, painless or normal
    combining form
    From Greek *eu* = well, from *eus* = good

euphoria	an exaggerated, irrational or groundless feeling of wellbeing
euploid	having an even multiple of all the chromosomes in a set
euthanasia	the act or practice of putting someone painlessly to death, especially in cases of incurable suffering

    ◑ Opposite ▸**dys-**

eversion
    the action of turning an organ or body part outwards or inside out
    noun
    From Latin *eversio* = overthrow, from *e* = out and *vertere* = to turn

ex- see ▸**e-, ex-; ec-, ex-**

exo-
    denoting outside, external
    combining form
    From Greek *exō* = out, outside

exocrine gland	a gland that secretes its products through a duct to the outside of the body
exoenzyme	an enzyme that functions outside the cell producing it
exotoxin	a toxin produced by a micro-organism and secreted into the surrounding medium

! Do not confuse with ▸ **e-, ex-; ec-, ex-; ecto-**
≈ Latin equivalent ▸ **extra-**
◐ Opposite ▸ **end-, endo-; ent-, ento-**

extra-
outside
combining form
From Latin ***extra*** = outside

| **extra**cellular | located or occurring outside the walls of a cell |
| **extra**uterine | located or developing outside the uterus |

≈ Greek equivalent ▸ **exo-**
◐ Opposite ▸ **intra-**

Ff

-facient
denoting causing, making or producing
combining form
From Latin ***faciens***, genitive ***facientis*** = doing, making, from ***facere*** = to do, to make

aborti**facient**	a drug or other means of causing abortion
febri**facient**	producing fever
rube**facient**	a substance applied to the skin that makes it redden, especially a counter-irritant

facio-
denoting the face
combining form
From Latin ***facies*** = face

faciolingual	relating to the face and tongue
facioplasty	reconstructive plastic surgery of the face
facioplegia	paralysis of the muscles of the face

faeco-
denoting faeces
combining form
From Latin ***faeces***, plural of ***faex*** = dregs, grounds

  faeco-oral transmission   the transmission of disease through contact of
                                        faecal matter with the mouth

≈ Greek equivalent ▸ **copr-, copro-**

fasci-, fascio-
denoting a sheath of connective tissue covering a muscle or organ
combining form
From Latin ***fascia*** = band, bandage

  fasciitis   inflammation of the fascia of a muscle or organ

fascia
a sheath of connective tissue covering a muscle or organ
noun
From Latin ***fascia*** = band, bandage
Plural form **fasciae**
◑ Related words **fascial** *adj* ▸ relating to a fascia

fascio- see ▸ fasci-, fascio-

fauces
the upper part of the throat, from the root of the tongue to the pharynx
noun
From Latin ***fauces*** = throat
◑ Related words **faucal** *or* **faucial** *adj* ▸ relating to the fauces

febri-
relating to fever
combining form
From Latin ***febris*** = fever

  febrifacient   producing fever
  febrifuge   a medicine or other agent that reduces fever

febrile
relating to fever
adjective
From medieval Latin ***febrilis***, from ***febris*** = fever

femora see ▸ femur

femoral

relating to the thigh
adjective
From Latin *femur*, genitive *femoris* = thigh

femoral artery   the main artery of the thigh

femur

the thigh bone
noun
From Latin *femur*, genitive *femoris* = thigh
Plural form **femora** (or **femurs**)

fenestra

an aperture in a bone or cartilage
noun
From Latin *fenestra* = opening in a wall, window
Plural form **fenestrae**

fenestra ovalis   an oval membrane-covered opening between the
                middle and the internal ear
fenestra rotunda   a round membrane-covered opening between the
                middle and the internal ear

-ferous

denoting bearing, producing, having or containing
combining form
From Latin *-fer* = bearing, carrying or bringing, from Latin *ferre* = to bear, to carry,
to bring

lacti**ferous**   conveying or producing milk or milky juice
mammi**ferous**   having breasts or milk glands
sangui**ferous**   conveying blood
somni**ferous**   inducing sleep

ferri-

denoting iron
combining form
From Latin *ferrum* = iron

ferritin   a protein in which iron is stored in the liver and spleen

≈ Greek equivalent ▸ **sider-, sidero-**

ferric

relating to or containing iron
adjective
From Latin ***ferrum*** = iron

fibr-, fibro-

denoting fibre or fibrous tissue
combining form
From Latin ***fibra*** = fibre

fibroblast	a cell in connective tissue from which fibrous tissue is formed
fibrocystic	relating to growth of fibrous tissue with cystic spaces
fibroma	a benign tumour composed of fibrous tissue
fibrosis	a pathological growth of fibrous tissue

fibula

the outer and thinner of the two bones extending from the knee to the ankle
noun
From Latin ***fibula*** = clasp, buckle, pin
Plural form **fibulae** (or **fibulas**)
◆ Related words **fibular** *adj* ▸relating to the fibula

-fic

denoting causing, making or producing
combining form
From Latin ***-ficus***, from ***facere*** = to do, to make

sopori**fic**	an agent that induces sleep
sudori**fic**	an agent that induces sweating

fistula

a narrow passage or duct between two hollow organs or between a hollow organ and the outer skin, occurring as a congenital abnormality or as a result of infection, injury or surgery
noun
From Latin ***fistula*** = pipe, tube, fistula
Plural form **fistulae** (or **fistulas**)
◆ Related words **fistular** *or* **fistulous** *adj* ▸relating to or resembling a fistula

flav-, flavi-, flavo-

denoting yellow
combining form
From Latin ***flavus*** = yellow

flavivirus   a virus of the Flaviridae family, which includes the virus responsible for yellow fever

foramen

a small opening, especially in a bone

noun

From Latin **foramen**, genitive **foraminis** = opening, from **forare** = to bore, to pierce

Plural form **foramina** (or **foramens**)

  foramen magnum   the large opening in the occipital bone through which the spinal cord joins the medulla oblongata

◆ Related words **foraminal** *adj* ▸relating to or consisting of a small opening, especially in a bone

-form

denoting a specified form or number of forms

combining form

From Latin **forma** = form, shape, appearance

  vermi**form**   worm-shaped

fornix

an arched structure

noun

From Latin **fornix**, genitive **fornicis** = arch, vault

Plural form **fornices**

  fornix cerebri   an arched structure formed by white matter in the brain

◆ Related words **fornical** *adj* ▸relating to or consisting of an arched structure

fossa

a depression

noun

From Latin **fossa** = ditch, trench

Plural form **fossae**

  iliac **fossa**   the depression in the ileum

fossula

a small depression

noun

From Latin **fossula** = little ditch, little trench

Plural form **fossulae**

◆ Related words **fossulate** *adj* ▸relating to or consisting of a small depression

fovea

a depression

noun

From Latin ***fovea*** = small pit

Plural form **foveae**

fovea centralis	a depression in the centre of the back of the retina, the place where vision is sharpest

◆ Related words **foveal** *adj* ▸ relating to a fovea

foveola

a small depression

noun

From new Latin ***foveola*** = very small pit, from Latin ***fovea*** = small pit

Plural form **foveolae**

fremitus

a vibration that can be felt by touching the body, especially the walls of the chest of someone speaking or coughing

noun

From Latin ***fremitus*** = roaring

Plural form **fremitus**

frontal

relating to the forehead; relating to the front part of an organ, body part, or body

adjective

From modern Latin ***frontalis***, from Latin ***frons***, genitive ***frontis*** = forehead, front

frontal bone	the bone that forms the forehead and the upper part of the eye sockets
frontal lobe	either of the two lobes of the brain behind the forehead

-fuge

denoting dispelling or expelling

combining form

From modern Latin ***-fugus***, from Latin ***fugare*** = to drive away, to chase away

febri**fuge**	a medicine or other agent that reduces fever
vermi**fuge**	a drug that expels worms from the intestine

-fusion

denoting pouring

combining form

From Latin ***fusum***, past participle of ***fundere*** = to pour

| per**fusion** | the passing of liquid through an organ or tissue |
| trans**fusion** | the passing of blood or blood products into the veins |

Gg

galact-, galacto-
denoting milk
combining form
From Greek *gala*, genitive *galaktos* = milk

galactorrhoea   excessive or inappropriate production of milk

≈ Latin equivalent ▸ **lact-, lacti-, lacto-**

galea
a structure or organ shaped like a helmet
noun
From Latin *galea* = helmet
Plural form **galeae**
◆ Related words **galeate** *adj* ▸relating to or consisting of a structure or organ shaped like a helmet

galei-, galeo-
denoting a helmet shape
combining form
From Latin *galea* = helmet

galeiform   shaped like a helmet

gam-, gamo-
denoting sexual union or sexual reproduction
combining form
From Greek *gamos* = marriage

gamete   a sexual reproductive cell such as an egg cell or sperm cell
gamogenesis   sexual reproduction

ganglion
a tumour in a tendon sheath (*pathol*); a nerve centre or a collection of nerve cells (*anat*)
noun
From Greek *ganglion* = encysted tumour on a tendon
Plural form **ganglia** (or **ganglions**)
◆ Related words **gangliar** *adj* ▸relating to a ganglion; **gangliate** *adj* ▸having a tumour in a tendon sheath (*pathol*) or having nerve centres (*anat*)

gastr-, gastro-
denoting the stomach or belly
combining form
From Greek **gastēr** = stomach, belly, womb

gastralgia	stomach pain
gastritis	inflammation of stomach lining
gastroenteritis	inflammation of the lining of the stomach and intestines
gastrointestinal	relating to or consisting of the stomach and intestines
gastrostomy	a surgical operation in which an opening is made in the stomach to introduce food into it

gastric
relating to or located in the stomach
adjective
From modern Latin **gastricus**, from Greek **gastēr** = stomach, belly, womb

gastric flu	any of several disorders of the stomach and intestinal tract, with symptoms of nausea, diarrhoea, abdominal cramps and fever
gastric juice	a thin clear acid fluid secreted by the stomach to effect digestion

gastro- see ▸ gastr-, gastro-

-gen
denoting something that produces something else; denoting something that is produced
combining form
From Greek **-genēs** = born, from **gignesthai** = to become, to be born

aller**gen**	any substance that induces an allergic reaction
andro**gen**	any of the male sex hormones that stimulate the development of male secondary sexual characteristics
anti**gen**	any substance that stimulates the production of an antibody

gene
the hereditary determinant of a specified difference between individuals, shown by molecular analysis to be a specific sequence or parts of a sequence of DNA
noun
From German **Gen**, from Greek **-genēs** = born, from **gignesthai** = to become, to be born

-genesis

denoting creation or development
combining form
From Greek **genesis** = origin, birth, production, generation, creation

patho**genesis**	the cause and development of a disease
spermato**genesis**	the production of sperm in the testes

-genic

denoting producing or produced by
combining form
From Greek **-genēs** = born, from **gignesthai** = to become, to be born

aller**genic**	producing an allergic reaction
carcino**genic**	capable of causing cancer
iatro**genic**	induced unintentionally in a patient by the treatment or comments of a physician
patho**genic**	producing disease

genio-

denoting the chin
combining form
From Greek **geneion** = chin

geniohyoid	relating to the chin and the hyoid bone
genioplasty	plastic surgery of the chin

! Do not confuse with ▸**geno-**

genital

relating to the sexual organs or to sexual reproduction
adjective
From Latin **genitalis** = relating to generation or birth, genital, from **gignere** = to father, to bear

genital herpes	a sexually transmitted skin disease on or around the sexual organs or anus, caused by a variety of the herpes simplex virus
genital wart	a wart on or around the sexual organs or anus, caused by a sexually transmitted disease

-genital

relating to the sexual organs or to sexual reproduction
combining form
From Latin **genitalis** = relating to generation or birth, genital, from **gignere** = to father, to bear

| anogenital | relating to the anus and the sexual organs |
| urogenital | relating to the urinary and sexual functions or organs |

genito-
denoting the sexual organs
combining form
From Latin **genitalis** = relating to generation or birth, genital, from **gignere** = to father, to bear

| **genito**-urinary | relating to the sexual and urinary functions or organs |

geno-
denoting genes
combining form
From Greek **genos** = race, offspring, class, kind

| **geno**type | the particular alleles at specified loci present in an individual; the genetic constitution; a group of individuals all of whom possess the same genetic constitution |

! Do not confuse with ▸**genio-**

genu
the knee; a bend or structure resembling a knee
noun
From Latin **genu** = knee
Plural form **genua**

| **genu** valgum | knock-knee |
| **genu** varum | bow legs |

◆ Related words **genual** *adj* ▸relating to the knee or to a bend or structure resembling a knee

ger-, gero-
denoting old age
combining form
From Greek **gēras** = old age

geriatrics	the medical care of the old
geroderma	the skin in old age
pro**ger**ia	a rare disease causing premature ageing in children

geront-, geronto-
denoting old age
combining form
From Greek **gerōn**, genitive **gerontos** = old man

| **geronto**logy | the scientific study of the processes of growing old |

gingiv-, gingivo-
denoting the gums
combining form
From Latin ***gingiva*** = gum

gingivectomy   the surgical removal of inflamed or excess gum

gingivitis   inflammation of the gums

gingival
relating to the gums
adjective
From Latin ***gingiva*** = gum

-globin
denoting a protein constituent
combining form
From Latin ***globus*** = ball, sphere, globe

haemo**globin**   a protein that carries oxygen in the blood

myo**globin**   a protein that stores oxygen in muscle

gloss-, glosso-
denoting the tongue
combining form
From Greek ***glōssa*** = tongue

glossodynia   pain in the tongue

glossopharyngeal   relating to the tongue and the pharynx

glossa
the tongue
noun
From Greek ***glōssa*** = tongue
Plural form **glossae** (or **glossas**)
◆ Related words **glossal** *adj* ▸relating to the tongue

glosso- see ▸ gloss-, glosso-

gluteal
relating to the buttocks or to the gluteus muscles of the buttock and hip area
adjective
From Greek ***gloutos*** = rump
≈ Latin equivalent ▸ **natal**[2]

-gluteal

denoting the buttocks or the gluteus muscles of the buttock and hip area

From Greek **gloutos** = rump

inter**gluteal**	between the buttocks
intra**gluteal**	within or into the gluteus muscles

glyc-, glyco-

denoting sugar or glucose

combining form

From Greek **glykys** = sweet

glycogen	a starch found in the liver and muscles that yields glucose on hydrolysis
glycolysis	the breakdown of glucose into acids, with the release of energy
hyper**glyc**aemia	an excessively high blood sugar level

gnathal see ▸ gnathic

-gnathia

denoting a condition in which the jaw is of a particular type

combining form

From Greek **gnathos** = jaw

a**gnathia**	a congenital condition in which the lower jaw is partially or completely absent
macro**gnathia**	abnormal largeness of the upper or lower jaw

gnathic, gnathal

relating to the jaw

adjective

From Greek **gnathos** = jaw

-gnosia

denoting knowledge or recognition

combining form

From Greek **gnōsis** = knowledge

a**gnosia**	an inability to recognize familiar things or people, especially after brain damage

-gnosis

denoting knowledge or recognition

combining form

From Greek **gnōsis** = knowledge

Plural form -**gnoses**

| di**gnosis** | the identification of a disease by means of its symptoms |
| pro**gnosis** | a forecast of the course of a disease |

-gnostic
denoting knowing or recognizing
combining form
From Greek **gnōstikos** = relating to knowledge, cognitive, from **gnōsis** = knowledge

| dia**gnostic** | relating to or useful in the identification of a disease by means of its symptoms |
| pro**gnostic** | relating to the forecasting of the course of a disease |

-gogue see ▶ -agogue

goni-, gonio-
denoting a corner or angle
combining form
From Greek **gōnia** = corner, angle

| **gonio**meter | an instrument for measuring angles |
| **gonio**scope | a viewing instrument for examining the corner between the iris and the cornea of the eye |

-gram
denoting something written or drawn to form a record
combining form
From Greek **gramma** = letter

| electrocardio**gram** | a photographic record of the electrical variations that occur during contraction of the muscle of the heart |
| encephalo**gram** | an X-ray photograph of the brain |

! Do not confuse with ▶ **-graph**

granul-, granulo-
denoting granules
combining form
From late Latin **granulum** = small grain, from Latin **granum** = grain

| **granulo**cyte | a white blood cell with granules in the protoplasm surrounding its nuleus |
| **granul**oma | a localized collection of macrophages or other inflammatory cells, caused by infection or invasion by a foreign body and having a granular appearance |

-graph

denoting a device that writes or records something; denoting something written or drawn to form a record

combining form

From Greek **graphē** = writing, drawing

    electrocardio**graph** an instrument for measuring electric currents, used for making photographic records of the electrical variations that occur during contraction of the muscle of the heart

    encephalo**graph**   an X-ray photograph of the brain

   ! Do not confuse with ▸**-gram**

gula

the upper part of the throat

noun

From Latin **gula** = throat

Plural form **gulae** (or **gulas**)

◆ Related words **gular** *adj* ▸relating to the upper part of the throat

gutta

a drop of medicine

noun

From Latin **gutta** = drop

Plural form **guttae**

Abbreviation **gt.**

◆ Related words **guttate** *adj* ▸resembling a drop or drops

gyn-, gynaeco-, gyno-

denoting woman, women, female, female sexual organs

combining form

From Greek **gynē**, genitive **gynaikos** = woman

    gynaecology   the scientific study of women's physiology and diseases

gyrus

a fold on the surface of the brain

noun

From Latin **gyrus** = circle, from Greek **gyros** = ring, circle

Plural form **gyri**

    dentate **gyrus**   a fold on the surface of the hippocampus

Hh

haem-, haemat-, haemato-, haemo-
denoting blood
combining form
From Greek *haima*, genitive *haimatos* = blood

haemagglutination the clumping together of red blood cells

haematogenesis   the formation of blood

haematoma   a swelling composed of blood effused into connective tissue

haemoglobin   a protein that carries oxygen in the blood

≈ Latin equivalent ▸**sangui-, sanguin-, sanguino-**

-halation
denoting breathing
combining form
From Latin *halare* = to breathe

in**halation**   breathing in

ex**halation**   breathing out

hallux
the big toe of a foot
noun
From modern Latin *hallux*, from Latin *allex*, *allus* or *hallus* = big toe
Plural form **halluces**

hamartoma
a non-cancerous mass comprising elements normally found in the tissue but in abnormal abundance and relation to each other
noun
From Greek *hamartia* = fault and *-ōma* = an ending of nouns formed from verbs with an infinitive ending in *-oun* (see ▸**-oma**)
Plural form **hamartomata** (or **hamartomas**)
◆ Related words **hamartomatous** *adj* ▸relating to a hamartoma

hapl-, haplo-
denoting single; denoting haploid
combining form
From Greek *haplous* = single, simple and *-oeidēs* = resembling, having the form of, from *eidos* = form, shape

| **hapl**oid | having a single set of unpaired chromosomes |
| **haplo**type | a set of alleles located on a single chromosome and inherited as a unit |

hapt-, hapto-
denoting combination, touch
combining form
From Greek ***haptein*** = to fasten, to join, to grasp, to touch

| **hapt**en | a substance, usually a small molecule, that can combine with an antibody but can initiate an immune response only when it is attached to a carrier molecule |
| **hapto**globin | a protein that combines with free haemoglobin in the blood and prevents its filtration through the kidney |

hemi-
denoting half
combining form
From Greek ***hēmi-*** = half-

hemialgia	pain confined to one side of the body
hemianopsia	blindness in half of the field of vision
hemiplegia	paralysis of one side of the body only
hemizygous	having only one representative of a gene or chromosome, as male mammals, which have only one X-chromosome

≈ Latin equivalent ▸ **demi-**; **semi-**

hepat-, hepato-
denoting the liver
combining form
From Latin ***hepar***, genitive ***hepatis***, from Greek ***hēpar***, genitive ***hēpatos*** = liver

| **hepato**cyte | a liver cell |
| **hepato**logy | the study of liver diseases |

hepatic
relating to or acting on the liver
adjective
From Latin ***hepaticus***, from Greek ***hēpatikos*** = relating to the liver

| **hepatic** vein | a vein draining blood from the liver into the inferior vena cava |

hepato- see ▸ hepat-, hepato-

heter-, hetero-

denoting other, different

combining form

From Greek **heteros** = other, different

heteroplasia	the development of abnormal tissue or tissue in an abnormal place
heteropsia	different vision in each eye
heterosexual	sexually attracted to persons of the opposite sex
heterozygous	having two different alleles of a gene

Opposite ▸ **homo-**

hiatus

a break, gap or opening

noun

From Latin **hiatus** = opening, aperture, cleft, from **hiare** = to open, to gape

Plural form **hiatus** (or **hiatuses**)

hiatus hernia	a hernia in which part of the stomach protrudes into the chest through a gap in the diaphragm

◆ Related words **hiatal** *adj* ▸ relating to a break, gap or opening

hidr-, hidro-

denoting sweat

combining form

From Greek **hidrōs** = sweat

hidropoiesis	the production of sweat
hidrosis	sweating, especially in excess

! Do not confuse with ▸ **hydr-, hydro-**

hilum

a depression or opening in an organ at the place where blood vessels, ducts, etc enter it

noun

From Latin **hilum** = trifle

Plural form **hila**

Alternative form **hilus** (*plural* **hili**)

histio-

denoting tissue

combining form

From Greek **histion** = web, cloth, sheet, sail

histiocyte	a macrophage that resides in the tissues of the body

histo-

denoting tissue
combining form
From Greek ***histos*** = web, warp

histamine	a pro-inflammatory amine molecule that is released from the tissues during an allergic response
histocompatibility	the factor determining the acceptance or rejection of cells
histology	the study of the microscopic structure of tissues and cells

hol-, holo-

denoting whole or wholly
combining form
From Greek ***holos*** = whole

holistic medicine	a form of medicine that considers the whole person, physically and psychologically, rather than treating merely the diseased or injured part
holocrine	producing a secretion of completely disintegrated cells

homeo-

denoting like, similar
combining form
From Greek ***homoios*** = like, similar, same

homeopathy	a type of alternative medicine, based on the principle of treating diseases with small quantities of drugs that produce symptoms similar to those of the disease
homeostasis	the tendency for the internal environment of the body to remain constant in spite of varying external conditions

! Do not confuse with ▸ **homo-**
◐ Opposite ▸ **allo-**; **heter-, hetero-**

homo-

denoting same
combining form
From Greek ***homos*** = same, common, joint

homograft	a graft of tissue from one individual to another of the same species
homosexual	sexually attracted to persons of the same sex
homozygous	having two identical alleles of a gene

! Do not confuse with ▸ **homeo-**

humeral

relating to the shoulder or the bone of the upper arm

adjective

From late Latin ***humeralis*** = relating to the upper arm or shoulder, from Latin ***umerus*** or ***humerus*** = upper arm, shoulder

! Do not confuse with ▸ **humoral**

humerus

the bone of the upper arm

noun

From Latin ***umerus*** or ***humerus*** = upper arm, shoulder

Plural form **humeri**

humoral

relating to or proceeding from a body fluid

adjective

From medieval Latin ***humoralis*** = relating to liquid, fluid or moisture, from Latin ***umor*** or ***humor*** = liquid, fluid, moisture

humoral immunity an acquired immunity in which antibodies circulating in body fluids play the major part

! Do not confuse with ▸ **humeral**

humour

a body fluid

noun

From Latin ***umor*** or ***humor*** = liquid, fluid, moisture

aqueous **humour**   the watery fluid between the cornea and the lens in the eye

vitreous **humour**   the jellylike substance filling the posterior chamber of the eye, between the lens and the retina

hyal-, hyalo-

relating to or resembling glass

combining form

From Greek ***hyalos*** = glass

hyaloid   glassy, clear or transparent

hyaloplasm   the clear fluid part of protoplasm

hyalophagia   a craving to eat glass

hydr-, hydro-

denoting water or fluid

combining form

From Greek *hydro-* = water-, from *hydōr* = water

de**hydr**ation	excessive loss of water from the tissues of the body
hydrocephalus	an abnormal accumulation of cerebrospinal fluid in the ventricles of the brain
hydrophobic	afraid of water (*psych*); repelling water (*biochem*)

! Do not confuse with ▸ **hidr-, hidro-**; **hygr-, hygro-**

hygiene
the preservation of health through cleanliness
noun
From Gr *hygieinē* (*technē*) hygienic (art), from *hygieia* health, from *hygiēs* healthy
◆ Related words **hygienic** *adj* ▸relating to hygiene
hygienist *n* a person skilled in hygiene, eg a dental hygienist

hygr-, hygro-
denoting wet, moist
combining form
From Greek *hygros* = wet, moist

hygroma	a swelling filled with fluid
hygrometer	an instrument for measuring the humidity of the air or of other gases

! Do not confuse with ▸ **hydr-, hydro-**

hymen
a membrane that partly covers the vaginal opening
noun
From Greek *hymēn* = membrane
◆ Related words **hymenal** *adj* ▸relating to the hymen

hyper-
denoting over, excessive, more than normal
combining form
From Greek *hyper* = over, beyond

hyperextend	to extend a limb beyond its normal range
hyperlipidaemia	an excessively high level of fat in the blood
hypertension	high blood pressure

! Do not confuse with ▸ **hyp-, hypo-**
≈ Latin equivalent ▸ **super-; supra-**

hyp-, hypo-

denoting under, defective, inadequate

combining form

From Greek **hypo** = under

hypoglycaemia	an excessively low blood sugar level
hypoplasia	underdevelopment
hypothalamus	a part of the brain that lies under the thalamus
hypoxia	a deficiency in the amount of oxygen reaching the body tissues

! Do not confuse with ▸ **hyper-**; **hypn-, hypno-**

≈ Latin equivalent ▸ **sub-**

hypn-, hypno-

denoting sleep; denoting hypnosis

combining form

From Greek **hypnos** = sleep

hypnagogic	relating to the period of drowsiness prior to sleep
hypnotherapy	the use of hypnosis eg in the management of pain or the treatment of psychosomatic disorders

! Do not confuse with ▸ **hyp-, hypo-**

≈ Latin equivalent ▸ **somn-, somni-, somno-**

Ii

-iasis

denoting a diseased condition

combining form

From Greek **-iasis** = denoting a state or condition

candid**iasis**	a yeast infection of the skin or mucous membranes
psor**iasis**	a skin disease characterized by red scaly pimples and patches

-iatric

denoting medical care or treatment within a particular speciality

combining form

From Greek **iatrikos** = relating to doctors, medical from **iatros** = doctor, physician from **iasthai** = to heal, to cure, to treat

paed**iatric**	relating to the medical treatment of children
pod**iatric**	relating to the medical treatment of disorders of the foot
psych**iatric**	relating to the medical treatment of diseases of the mind

iatro-
denoting a doctor, physician, or medical treatment
combining form
From Greek *iatros* = doctor, physician, from *iasthai* = to heal, to cure, to treat
   iatrogenic   induced unintentionally in a patient by the treatment or comments of a physician

-id
denoting relationship
combining form
From Greek *-is*, genitive *-idos* = a suffix forming nouns and adjectives denoting relationship
   chromat**id**   one of the two thread-like structures formed by the longitudinal division of a chromosome

idio-
denoting peculiarity, particularity, separateness, isolation
combining form
From Greek *idios* = own, private, personal, separate
   idiopathic   arising spontaneously from some unknown cause
   idiotype   the specificity of an antibody, determining which antigen it will bind

-iferous see ▸ -ferous

ile-, ileo-
denoting the ileum
combining form
From Latin *ile*, *ileum* or *ilium* = groin, flank
   ileitis   inflammation of the ileum
   ileostomy   a surgical operation in which the ileum is brought through an artificial opening in the abdominal wall through which the contents of the intestine may be discharged

  ! Do not confuse with ▸ **ili-, ilio-**

ileum
the lowest part of the small intestine, between the jejunum and the caecum
noun
From Latin *ile*, *ileum* or *ilium* = groin, flank
Plural form **ilea**
  ! Do not confuse with ▸ **ilium**
  ◆ Related words **ileac** *or* **ileal** *adj* ▸ relating to the ileum

ili-, ilio-

denoting the ilium

combining form

From Latin *ile*, *ileum* or *ilium* = groin, flank

iliococcygeal   relating to the ilium and the coccyx

! Do not confuse with ▸ **ile-, ileo-**

ilium

a wide bone that is fused with the ischium and pubis to form the hip bone

noun

From Latin *ile*, *ileum* or *ilium* = groin, flank

Plural form **ilia**

! Do not confuse with ▸ **ileum**

◆ Related words **iliac** *adj* ▸ relating to the ilium

im-, in-, ir-

denoting not; denoting in, into

combining form

From Latin *in* = in, into; not

imperforate   lacking an opening, especially as a result of abnormal development

implant   something implanted in body tissue, such as a graft, a pellet containing a hormone, an artificial pacemaker, etc

infertile   not capable of producing offspring

inhalation   the act of drawing air or gas into the lungs; something to be drawn into the lungs

irradiation   the therapeutic application of electromagnetic radiation

irreducible   unable to be replaced in a normal position by manipulation, as a hernia, dislocation etc

immun-, immuno-

denoting the immune system, the system that protects the body from foreign or harmful organisms or substances

combining form

From Latin *immunis* = exempt, from Latin *in-* = not and *munis* = serving

immunize   to protect against an infection by stimulating the immune system with a vaccine

immunodeficient   failing to make a normal or adequate immune response

immunoglobulin   any of the proteins of the immune system that function as antibodies

infarct or infarction

an area of necrosis within a tissue, resulting from local ischaemia caused by
an obstruction of blood flow to the area

noun

From medieval Latin ***infarctus*** = forced in, from ***in*** = in and ***far(c)tus***, past
participle of ***farcire*** = to cram or stuff

inferior

lower, especially in position

adjective

From Latin ***inferior*** = lower, comparative form of ***inferus*** = situated underneath,
lower

    inferior vena cava   a vein that returns blood to the heart from the lower
                                    body

◑ Opposite ▸ **superior**

infra-

below

combining form

From Latin ***infra*** = below

    infracostal   beneath the ribs

    inframaxillary   situated under the jaw; belonging to the lower jaw

    infraorbital   situated below the orbit of the eye

! Do not confuse with ▸ **intra-**

◑ Opposite ▸ **supra-**

infundibulum

a funnel or funnel-shaped part, especially the funnel-shaped stalk that
connects the pituitary to the brain, the conical outflow portion of the right
ventricle of the heart, or a funnel-shaped passage where a calyx connects to
the renal pelvis

noun

From Latin ***infundibulum*** = funnel, from ***infundere*** = to pour in

Plural form **infundibula**

◆ Related words **infundibular** *adj* ▸ having or shaped like a funnel

infundiform *adj* ▸ funnel-shaped

ino-

denoting fibrous tissue or muscle

combining form

From Greek ***is***, genitive ***inos*** = sinew, tendon, fibrous muscle vessels

    inotropic   affecting or controlling muscular contraction, especially
                           in the heart

insula

a small lobe of the cerebrum hidden in the fissure of Sylvius (also called Reil's island)

noun

From Latin ***insula*** = island

Plural form **insulae**

inter-

denoting between, among, in the midst of, mutual, reciprocal, together

combining form

From Latin ***inter*** = between, among, in the midst of

interdental	between the teeth
intercostal muscles	the muscles between the ribs
intercellular signalling	signalling between cells

! Do not confuse with ▸**intra-**

interstice

a small space between things set close together, or between parts of the body

noun

From Latin ***interstitium*** = intervening space, interval, from ***intersistere*** = to stand in between

✦ Related words **interstitial** *adj* ▸relating to, occurring in or forming the small spaces between things set close together, or between parts of the body

intra-

within

combining form

From Latin ***intra*** = within, inside

intra-abdominal	within the cavity of the abdomen
intramedullary	within the bone marrow
intravenous	within or introduced into a vein or veins

! Do not confuse with ▸**infra-**; **inter-**; **intro-**

≈ Greek equivalent ▸**end-, endo-**; **ent-, ento-**

◑ Opposite ▸**extra-**

intro-

within, into

combining form

From Latin ***intro*** = inwardly, internally, to the inside

intromission the insertion of an organ or body part into another, especially of the penis into the vagina

in utero
in the womb
adjective, adverb
From Latin **in utero** = in the womb, from **in** = in and **uterus** = womb

inversion
the action of turning in an organ or body part, or of turning it inside out; a mutation of chromosomes in which certain genes are in reverse order
noun
From Latin **inversio** = inversion, from **invertere** = to turn upside down, from **in** = in and **vertere** = to turn

in vitro
occurring in a test tube
adjective, adverb
From Latin **in vitro** = in glass, from **in** = in and **vitrum** = glass
in vitro fertilization the fertilization of an ovum by mixing it with sperm in a culture medium, after which the fertilized egg implanted in the uterus to continue normal development

in vivo
occurring in a living organism
adjective, adverb
From Latin **in vivo** = in a living thing, from **in** = in and **vivum** = living thing, from **vivus** = alive, living

ir- see ▸ im-, in-, ir-

irid-, irido-
denoting the iris of the eye
combining form
From Greek **iris**, genitive **iridos** = rainbow, halo, iris
iridectomy the surgical removal of part of the iris
iridotomy a surgical incision into the iris of the eye

isch-
denoting deficiency, suppression or retention
combining form
From Greek **ischein** = to keep back, to restrain, to hold

isch**a**emia	an inadequate flow of blood to a part of the body
isch**u**ria	a reduction or stoppage of urine flow

ischium

a posterior bone of the pelvic girdle

noun

From Latin *ischium*, from Greek *ischion* = hip joint

Plural form **ischia**

◆ Related words **ischiadic**, **ischial** *or* **ischiatic** *adj* ▸relating to the ischium

iso-

denoting equal, equally, similar

combining form

From Greek *isos* = equal

isoenzyme	one of several variants of the same enzyme occurring within a single species
isomer	a substance that has the same composition as another but differs in structure
isomorphous	similar in shape or structure
isotonic solution	a solution that has the same osmotic pressure as another

isthmus

a narrow part of a structure connecting two larger parts

noun

From Latin *isthmus*, from Greek *isthmos* = neck, narrow passage

Plural form **isthmi** (or **isthmuses**)

-itis

denoting inflammation

combining form

From Greek *-itis* = feminine adjective ending agreeing with *nosos* = disease

appendic**itis**	inflammation of the appendix
laryng**itis**	inflammation of the larynx
rhin**itis**	inflammation of the mucous membrane of the nose
tendon**itis**	inflammation of a tendon

Jj

jejun-, jejuno-
denoting the part of the small intestine between the duodenum and the ileum

combining form

From Latin **jejunus** = fasting (because the jejunum is usually empty after death)

jejunectomy	the surgical removal of all or part of the jejunum
jejunoileal	relating to the jejunum and the ileum

jejunum
the part of the small intestine between the duodenum and the ileum

noun

From Latin **jejunus** = fasting (because it is usually empty after death)

◆ Related words **jejunal** *adj* ▸relating to the jejunum

juxta-
near to, next to, adjacent to

combining form

From Latin **iuxta** = near to, next to

juxta-articular	adjacent to a joint
juxta-epiphyseal	adjacent to an epiphysis

Kk

kal-
denoting potassium

combining form

From modern Latin **kalium** = potassium

hyper**kal**aemia	an abnormally high level of potassium in the blood
hypo**kal**aemia	an abnormally low level of potassium in the blood

kary-, karyo-
denoting the nucleus of a cell

combining form

From Greek **karyon** = nut, kernel

karyokinesis	the division of the nucleus of a cell during mitosis
karyotype	the appearance, number and arrangement of the chromosomes in the cells of an individual; a diagram or photograph of the chromosomes of a cell or cells

karyon

the nucleus of a cell

noun

From Greek ***karyon*** = nut, kernel

Plural form **karya** (or **karyons**)

kerat-, kerato-

denoting keratin or horny tissue; denoting the cornea

combining form

From Greek ***keras***, genitive ***keratos*** = horn

keratitis	inflammation of the cornea
keratosis	a horny growth on or over the skin, eg a wart; a skin condition producing this

keratin

a nitrogenous compound that is the main ingredient in nails, hair, and the outer skin layers

noun

From Greek ***keras***, genitive ***keratos*** = horn

kerato- see ▸ kerat-, kerato-

kil-, kilo-

denoting a thousand

combining form

From Greek ***chilioi*** = thousand

kilocalorie	1000 calories, a Calorie, used to measure the energy content of food

kin-, kine-, kines-, kinesi-, kinesio-

denoting movement

combining form

From Greek ***kinēsis*** = motion, movement, from ***kinein*** = to move

kinaesthesia	a sense of the body's movement or of muscular effort
kinesiology	the study of human movement and posture, including aspects of anatomy, biomechanics and physiology; any of various therapies that use gentle finger pressure to detect blockages and other physical problems as part of a holistic approach to treating disease

-kine

denoting movement

combining form

From Greek ***kinein*** = to move

cyto**kine**   a protein chemical messenger that assists the immune system in combating infection

---

kines-, kinesi- see ▸ **kin-, kine-, kines-, kinesi-, kinesio-**

-kinesia

denoting movement

combining form

From Greek ***kinēsis*** = motion, movement, from ***kinein*** = to move

a**kinesia**   the lack, loss or impairment of the power of voluntary movement

dys**kinesia**   a lack of control over bodily movements; impaired performance of voluntary movements

---

kinesio- see ▸ **kin-, kine-, kines-, kinesi-, kinesio-**

-kinesis

denoting movement

combining form

From Greek ***kinēsis*** = motion, movement, from ***kinein*** = to move

dia**kinesis**   the final stage of the first phase of meiosis, during which pairs of homologous chromosomes almost completely separate

---

-kinetic

denoting movement

combining form

From Greek ***kinētikos*** = relating to putting in motion, from ***kinein*** = to move

hyper**kinetic**   relating to abnormal movement in muscle or to hyperactivity

pharmaco**kinetic**   relating to the way the body deals with drugs

---

koil-, koilo-

denoting hollow or concave

combining form

From Greek ***koilos*** = hollow

koilocyte   a hollow or concave cell

koilonychia   a condition associated with iron-deficiency anaemia in which the fingernails are hollow and thin

kymo-
denoting a wave, oscillation
combining form
From Greek **kyma** = wave

kymograph	an instrument for recording the pressure of fluids, especially of blood in a blood vessel

kyph-, kypho-
denoting bent or curved forwards
combining form
From Greek **kyphos** = bent forwards, stooping, hunchbacked

kyphosis	a hunchbacked condition
kyphoscoliosis	a condition in which the spine is abnormally bent forwards and to the side

labi-, labio-
denoting the lips
combining form
From Latin **labium** = lip

labioglossolaryn-geal	relating to the lips, tongue and larynx
labioplasty	plastic surgery of a lip

≈ Greek equivalent ▸ **cheil-, cheilo-**

labial
relating to the lips; relating to the folds of skin surrounding the vaginal orifice in women
adjective
From medieval Latin **labialis**, from Latin **labium** = lip

labio- see ▸ **labi-, labio-**

labium
one of the folds of skin surrounding the vaginal orifice in women
noun
From Latin **labium** = lip
Plural form **labia**

| **labia** majora | the two larger outer folds of skin surrounding the vaginal orifice in women |
| **labia** minora | the two smaller inner folds of skin surrounding the vaginal orifice in human females |

lacrimal, lachrymal, lacrymal
relating to tears or the secretion of tears
adjective
From medieval Latin *lachrymalis*, from Latin *lacrima* = tear

| **lacrimal** duct | a duct that conveys tear water from the inner corner of the eye to the nose |
| **lacrimal** gland | a gland at the outer angle of the eye that secretes tears |

lact-, lacti-, lacto-
denoting milk
combining form
From Latin *lac*, genitive *lactis* = milk

lactiferous	conveying or producing milk or milky juice
lactogenic	inducing lactation
lactose	milk sugar

≈ Greek equivalent ▸ **galact-, galacto-**

lacuna
a cavity or depression, especially in a bone
noun
From Latin *lacuna* = pool, cavity, gap
Plural form **lacunae** (or **lacunas**)

laev-, laevo-, lev-, levo-
denoting on or to the left
combining form
From Latin *laevus* = left

| **laevo**cardia | the normal condition in which the heart lies in the left side of the chest |
| **laevo**rotatory | counter-clockwise; rotating the plane of polarization of light to the left |

◑ Opposite ▸ **dextr-, dextro-**

-lalia
denoting speech or a speech problem
combining form
From Greek *lalia* = talk, chat, from *lalein* = to talk, to chat, to chatter

| copro**lalia** | obsessive or repetitive use of obscene language, eg as a characteristic of Tourette's syndrome |
| echo**lalia** | the senseless or compulsive repetition of words heard, occurring in forms of mental illness |

lamina
a thin plate of bone or layer of tissue

noun

From Latin ***lamina*** = thin plate or layer

Plural form **laminae** (or **laminas**)

| **lamina** propria | a layer of connective tissue underneath the epithelium of an organ |

lapar-, laparo-
denoting the abdomen or the loins

combining form

From Greek ***lapara*** = flank

| **laparo**scopy | a surgical examination by means of a tube-shaped optical instrument which permits examination of the internal organs from outside |
| **laparo**tomy | the surgical cutting of the abdominal wall |

-lapaxy
denoting removal

combining form

From Greek ***lapaxis*** = evacuation, from ***lapattein*** = to empty, to evacuate

| litho**lapaxy** | the operation of crushing stone in the bladder and working it out |

laryng-, laryngo-
denoting the larynx

combining form

From Greek ***larynx***, genitive ***laryngos*** = larynx

| **laryng**ectomy | the surgical removal of the larynx |
| **laryngo**scope | a mirror for examining the larynx and trachea |

larynx
the upper part of the windpipe

noun

From Greek ***larynx***, genitive ***laryngos*** = larynx

Plural form **larynges** (or **larynxes**)

◆ Related words **laryngal** *or* **laryngeal** *adj* ▸ relating to the larynx

lateral

relating to, located on or affecting a side or sides

adjective

From Latin ***lateralis*** = of or on the side, lateral, from ***latus***, genitive ***lateris*** = side

-lateral

denoting a side

combining form

From Latin ***lateralis*** = of or on the side, lateral, from ***latus***, genitive ***lateris*** = side

bi**lateral**   relating to, located on or affecting both sides of the body or of an organ, or both of a pair of organs, each of which is located on a side of the body

lecithin

any of a group of complex phospholipids that are an important component of biological membranes, found in the yolk of an egg, in the brain, blood, etc

noun

From Greek ***lekithos*** = egg yolk

leio-

denoting smooth

combining form

From Greek ***leios*** = smooth

leiodermia   a condition in which the skin is abnormally smooth

leiomyoma   a benign tumour of smooth muscle, usually occurring in the uterus

-lemma

denoting membrane

combining form

From Greek ***lemma*** = rind, husk

Plural form **-lemmata** (or **-lemmas**)

axo**lemma**   the cell membrane enclosing the protoplasm of an axon

sarco**lemma**   the cell membrane enclosing a muscle fibre

-lepsy

denoting seizure

combining form

From Greek ***lēpsis*** = taking, seizing, seizure, from ***lambanein*** = to take, to seize

cata**lepsy**   a state where someone is more or less completely incapacitated, with bodily rigidity, as in hypnotic trances and sometimes in schizophrenia

| epi**lepsy** | a chronic functional disease of the nervous system, characterized by recurring attacks of sudden unconsciousness or impairment of consciousness, commonly accompanied by convulsive seizures |
| narco**lepsy** | a condition marked by short attacks of irresistible drowsiness |

-leptic
denoting seizure
combining form
From Greek **lēpsis** = taking, seizing, seizure, from **lambanein** = to take, to seize

| narco**leptic** | relating to or affected by short attacks of irresistible drowsiness |

lept-, lepto-
denoting slender, narrow, thin, small, slight
combining form
From Greek **leptos** = fine, small, thin, delicate, narrow, slight

| **lepto**cephalic | having a narrow head |
| **lepto**tene | the first stage of the prophase of meiosis in which long, slender, single-stranded chromosomes appear |

lepto- see ▸ lept-

leuc-, leuco-, leuk-, leuko-
denoting white; denoting leucocytes
combining form
From Greek **leukos** = white

leucocyte	a white blood cell
leucoderma	a condition in which white patches, surrounded by a pigmented area, appear in the skin
leucorrhoea	an abnormal discharge of whitish mucus or mucus and pus from the vagina
leukaemia	a cancerous disease in which too many white blood cells accumulate in the body

lev-, levo- see ▸ laev-, laevo-, lev-, levo-

-lexia
denoting reading
combining form
From Greek **lexis** = speech, word, as a result of confusion of Greek **legein** = to speak with Latin **legere** = to read

| a**lexia** | the loss of the ability to read |
| dys**lexia** | difficulty in learning to read or spell |

lien-, lieno-

denoting the spleen

combining form

From Latin **lien** = spleen

| **lieno**-intestinal | relating to the spleen and the intestines |
| **lieno**pathy | a disease of the spleen |

ligament

a bundle of fibrous tissue joining bones or cartilages

noun

From Latin **ligamentum** = band, tie, bandage, from **ligare** = to tie, to bind

ligate

to tie up a blood vessel, duct, artery, etc using a cord

verb

From Latin **ligatus** = tied, bound, from **ligare** = to tie, to bind

◆ Related words **ligation** *n* the action of tying up a blood vessel, duct, artery, etc

ligature

a cord used in surgery for tying up a blood vessel, duct, artery, etc

noun

to tie up a blood vessel, duct, artery, etc using a cord

verb

From Latin **ligatura** = band, ligature, from **ligare** = to tie, to bind

limbic

relating to or located at the edge of an organ or part; relating to the limbic system

adjective

From Latin **limbus** = edge

| **limbic** system | the system of nerves and networks in the brain, the hypothalamus, etc concerned with basic emotions |

limbus

the edge of an organ or part

noun

From Latin **limbus** = edge

Plural form **limbi**

| **limbus** sclerae | the part of the eye where the cornea meets the sclera |

limen

a boundary area (*anat*); the threshold of consciousness below which a stimulus is not perceived (*psychol*)

noun

From Latin *limen*, genitive *liminis* = threshold

Plural form **limina** (or **limens**)

    limen nasi   the part of the nasal cavity where bone meets cartilage

◆ Related words **liminal** *adj* ▸relating to a boundary area (*anat*); relating to the threshold of consciousness below which a stimulus is not perceived (*psychol*)

linea

a line or narrow strip

noun

From Latin *linea* = string, line

Plural form **lineae**

    linea alba   the line of tendon to which the abdominal muscles are attached that runs down the body from the bottom of the chest to the pubic bone

lip-, lipo-

denoting fat

combining form

From Greek *lipos* = fat

    lipaemia   an excess of fat in the blood

    lipogenesis   the formation of fat in the body

    lipoma   a fatty tumour

    liposuction   a surgical process for the removal of excess, unwanted fat from the body by suction

≈ Latin equivalent ▸ **adipo-**

lith-, litho-

denoting stone or calculus (a stone-like deposit or mass)

combining form

From Greek *lithos* = stone

    lithotomy   a surgical operation in which a stone is removed from an organ, especially the bladder

    litholapaxy   the operation of crushing a stone in the bladder and working it out

locus

an area or region (*anat*); the position of a gene on a chromosome (*genet*)

noun

From Latin **locus** = place
Plural form **loci**
   locus caeruleus   a blue area in the fourth ventricle of the brain

log-, logo-
denoting word, speech
combining form
From Greek **logos** = word, speech
   logagraphia   the loss of the ability to express ideas in writing as a result of brain injury
   logorrhoea   uncontrolled or incoherent talkativeness

-logy
denoting study, science
combining form
From Greek **-logia**, from **logos** = word, speech, subject
   epidemio**logy**   the study of epidemics and their occurrence, severity, distribution, etc
   histopatho**logy**   the study of the effects of disease on the tissues of the body
   nephro**logy**   the study of the structure, functions and diseases of the kidneys
   physio**logy**   the study of the processes of life in animals and plants

lord-, lordo-
denoting bent or curved backwards
combining form
From Greek **lordos** = bent backwards
   lordosis   a condition in which the spine is abnormally bent backwards

lumbar
relating to the section of the spine between the lowest rib and the pelvis
adjective
From medieval Latin **lumbaris**, from **lumbus** = loin
   lumbar puncture   the insertion of a needle into the lower part of the spinal cord to take a specimen of cerebrospinal fluid, inject drugs, etc

lumen
the cavity of a tubular organ
noun
From Latin **lumen**, genitive **luminis** = light, opening

Plural form **lumina** (or **lumens**)

◆ Related words **lumenal** or **luminal** adj ▸relating to the cavity of a tubular organ

luteal

relating to the corpus luteum or its formation

adjective

From Latin **luteus** = yellow, referring to the yellow colour of the corpus luteum

luteo-

denoting yellow; denoting the corpus luteum

combining form

From Latin **luteus** = yellow, referring to the yellow colour of the corpus luteum

luteinization	the stimulation of the ovary, whereby ovulation occurs and a corpus luteum is formed

lymph

a colourless or faintly yellowish fluid containing white blood cells that is collected into the lymphatic vessels from body tissues

noun

From Latin **lympha** = water

lymph node or gland	any of the small masses of tissue sited along the lymphatic vessels, in which lymph is purified, and lymphocytes are formed

lymph-, lympho-

denoting lymph or the lymphatic system

combining form

From Latin **lympha** = water

lymphadenopathy	a disease of the lymph nodes
lymphangial	relating to the lymphatic vessels
lymphocyte	a small white blood cell, one of many present in lymphoid tissues, circulating in blood and lymph and involved in antigen-specific immune reactions
lymphoma	a tumour consisting of lymphoid tissue

-lysis

denoting the action of loosening, breaking down or dividing into parts.

combining form

From Greek **lysis** = releasing, loosening, dissolution, from **luein** = to release, to loosen, to dissolve

glyco**lysis**	the breakdown of glucose into acids, with the release of energy

haemo**lysis**	the breaking up of red blood cells
para**lysis**	a loss of power of motion or sensation in any part of the body

Mm

macr-, macro-

denoting large, especially abnormally large

combining form

From Greek ***makros*** = long, large

macrencephaly	abnormal largeness of the brain
macrocephaly	abnormal largeness of the head
macrocyte	an abnormally large red blood cell associated with some forms of anaemia
macrophage	any of the large phagocytic cells sited in the walls of blood vessels and found in connective tissue, usually immobile but stimulated into mobility by inflammation

macul-, maculo-

denoting a discoloured area on the skin; denoting the small yellow area at the centre of the retina at which vision is most distinct

combining form

From Latin ***macula*** = spot, mark, stain

maculopapular	characterized by maculae and papules
maculopathy	a disease of the macula lutea

macula

a discoloured area on the skin; the small yellow area at the centre of the retina at which vision is most distinct

noun

From Latin ***macula*** = spot, mark, stain

Plural form **maculae**

macula lutea	the small yellow area at the centre of the retina at which vision is most distinct

macular

relating to or consisting of a discoloured area or areas on the skin; relating to the small yellow area at the centre of the retina at which vision is most distinct

adjective

From Latin ***macula*** = spot, mark, stain

maculo-

macular degeneration   degeneration of the macula lutea, which causes loss of central vision

maculo- see ▸ **macul-, maculo-**

mal-
denoting bad, badly, wrong, wrongly, abnormal or defective
combining form
From Latin ***male*** = badly

malabsorption   poor absorption of one or more nutrients by the small intestine, a symptom of coeliac disease, cystic fibrosis, etc

malformation   deformity

malnutrition   inadequate or faulty nutrition

malocclusion   imperfect positioning of the upper and lower teeth when the jaw is closed

-malacia
denoting softening
combining form
From Greek ***malakia*** = softness

kerato**malacia**   the softening of the cornea, resulting from a deficiency of vitamin A

osteo**malacia**   the softening of bones by absorption of their calcium salts, resulting from a deficiency of vitamin D

mamm-, mammi-, mammo-
denoting female breasts or milk glands
combining form
From Latin ***mamma*** = breast

mammectomy   the surgical removal of a breast

mammiferous   having breasts or milk glands

mammogram   an X-ray photograph of the breast

mammoplasty   plastic surgery to change the shape of the breasts, as by the use of silicone implants, etc

mammary
relating to female breasts or milk glands
adjective
From Latin ***mamma*** = breast

mammary gland   a gland in the female breast that produces milk

mammi-, mammo- see ▸ **mamm-, mammi-, mammo-**

mandible

a jaw or jawbone, especially the lower jaw or jawbone

noun

From Latin ***mandibula*** = jaw, from ***mandere*** = to chew

◆ Related words **mandibular** *adj* ▸relating to a jaw or jawbone, especially the lower jaw or jawbone

mania

a mental illness characterized by euphoria, excessively rapid speech and violent, destructive actions; the elated phase of manic-depressive or bipolar psychosis

noun

From Latin ***mania*** = madness, from Greek ***mania*** = madness

◆ Related words **manic** *adj* ▸relating to or affected by mania

manus

a hand

noun

From Latin ***manus*** = hand

Plural form **manus**

◆ Related words **manual** *adj* ▸relating to the hands

mast-, masto-

denoting a breast or milk gland

combining form

From Greek ***mastos*** = breast

mastectomy	the surgical removal of a breast
mastitis	inflammation of the breast
mastodynia	pain in the breasts
mastopathy	a disease of the milk glands

maxill-, maxilli-, maxillo-

denoting a jawbone, especially the upper jawbone

combining form

From Latin ***maxilla*** = jawbone, jaw

maxillodental	relating to the upper jaw and upper set of teeth
maxillofacial	relating to the jawbone and face

maxilla

a jawbone, especially the upper jawbone

noun

From Latin ***maxilla*** = jawbone, jaw

Plural form **maxillae**

◆ Related words **maxillary** *adj* ▸relating to a jawbone, especially the upper jawbone

---

maxilli-, maxillo- see ▸ **maxill-, maxilli-, maxillo-**

---

meat-, meato-

denoting an opening of a passage or canal

combining form

From Latin **meatus** = passage, from **meare** = to go, to pass

meatoplasty	plastic surgery of a passage or canal
meatoscope	a viewing instrument for examining a passage or canal, especially the urethra
meatotomy	a surgical incision into the opening of the urethra

---

meatus

an opening of a passage or canal

noun

From Latin **meatus** = passage, from **meare** = to go, to pass

Plural form **meatus** (or **meatuses**)

◆ Related words **meatal** *adj* ▸relating to an opening of a passage or canal

---

medial

relating to or located in the middle; located near the median plane of the body or an organ

adjective

From Latin **medialis** = middle, from **medius** = middle

---

median

relating to or located in the plane that divides the body or an organ into left and right halves

adjective

From Latin **medianus** = middle, from **medius** = middle

---

medulla

the inner portion of an organ, hair, or tissue; bone marrow; a medulla oblongata

noun

From Latin **medulla** = marrow

Plural form **medullae** (or **medullas**)

medulla oblongata the part of the brain that tapers off into the spinal cord

mega-

denoting large, especially abnormally large; denoting one million
combining form
From Greek *megas*, genitive *megalou* = large, great

megacephalous	having an abnormally large head
megadose	a very large dose of a medicine or drug
megajoule	one million joules

megal-, megalo-

denoting large, especially abnormally large, or great
combining form
From Greek *megas*, genitive *megalou* = large, great

megaloblast	an abnormally large nucleated red blood cell found in the bone marrow of people with some forms of anaemia
megalomania	the delusion that one is great or powerful

-megaly

denoting largeness or enlargement, especially abnormal largeness or enlargement
combining form
From Greek *megas*, genitive *megalou* = large, great

cardio**megaly**	abnormal enlargement of the heart
spleno**megaly**	abnormal enlargement of the spleen

mei-, meio-

denoting reduction
combining form
From Greek *meiōn* = less, lesser

meiocyte	a cell that divides by meiosis
meiosis	a type of cell division by which the chromosomes are reduced from the diploid to the haploid number during the formation of gametes

melan-, melano-

denoting black or dark; denoting melanin
combining form
From Greek *melas*, genitive *melanos* = black, dark

melanin	the dark pigment in skin, hair, etc
melanocyte	an epidermal cell that can produce melanin
melanoma	any skin tumour consisting of melanin-pigmented cells
melanuria	the presence of a dark pigment in the urine

-melia

denoting a condition in which the limbs are of the specified type
combining form
From Greek **melos** = limb

a**melia**	a congenital condition in which one or more limbs are completely absent
dys**melia**	a condition in which one or more limbs are misshapen or incomplete

men-, meno-

denoting menstruation
combining form
From Greek **mēn**, genitive **mēnos** = month

menarche	the first menstruation
menopause	the ending of menstruation
menorrhagia	an excessive flow of blood during menstruation
menorrhea	a normal flow of blood during menstruation

mening-, meningo-

denoting the meninges of the brain
combining form
From Greek **mēninx**, genitive **mēningos** = membrane

meningitis	inflammation of the meninges
meningocele	a protrusion of the meninges through the skull or spine
meningococcus	a spherical bacterium which causes epidemic cerebrospinal meningitis

meninges

the three membranes that envelop the brain and spinal cord
noun
From Greek **mēninges**, plural of **mēninx**, genitive **mēningos** = membrane
Singular form **meninx**
◆ Related words **meningeal** *adj* ▸relating to the meninges

meninx see ▸ meninges

mental[1]

relating to the mind
adjective
From late Latin **mentalis** = mental, from Latin **mens**, genitive **mentis** = mind

mental²

relating to the chin

adjective

From Latin **mentum** = chin

-mentia

denoting mental powers

combining form

From Latin **mens**, genitive **mentis** = mind

a**mentia**   a failure to develop mentally

de**mentia**   any form of insanity characterized by the failure or loss of mental powers; the organic deterioration of intelligence, memory, and orientation in advancing age

-mere

denoting a part

combining form

From Greek **meros** = part

blasto**mere**   a cell produced by cleavage of a fertilized ovum in the earliest stages of embryonic development

centro**mere**   the portion of a chromosome that attaches to the spindle during cell division

telo**mere**   the structure which terminates the arm of a chromosome, protecting the chromosome against gene loss and decay

mes-, meso-

denoting middle, medium, or intermediate

combining form

From Greek **mesos** = middle

mesencephalon   the mid-brain

mesocephalic   having a medium-sized head

mesoderm   the layer of embryonic cells between the ectoderm and the endoderm in a gastrula

mesogastrium   the region of the abdomen between the epigastrium and the hypogastrium

met-, meta-

denoting beyond; denoting change

combining form

From Greek **meta** = among, with, after, beyond

metacarpus   the part of the hand between the wrist and the fingers, ie beyond the wrist

metastasis the transfer of disease from its original site to another part of the body; a secondary tumour distant from the original site of disease

metr-, metro-
denoting the uterus
combining form
From Greek ***mētra*** = womb

endo**metr**iosis the presence of active endometrial tissue where it should not be, especially when affecting other organs of the pelvic cavity

metrorrhagia bleeding from the uterus between menstrual periods

micr-, micro-
denoting small, especially abnormally small; denoting a microscope; denoting one millionth
combining form
From Greek ***mikros*** = small

micrognathia abnormal smallness of one or both jaws

microgram one millionth of a gram

micrurgy the technique of using delicate instruments to work on cells, bacteria, etc, under high magnifications

milium
a whitish pimple formed on the skin, usually by a clogged sebaceous gland
noun
From Latin ***milium*** = millet
Plural form **milia**

miliary
characterized by small skin eruptions resembling millet seed
adjective
From Latin ***miliarius*** = relating to millet, from ***milium*** = millet

miliary a form of tuberculosis characterized by small nodules
tuberculosis resembling millet seeds

milli-
denoting a thousandth
combining form
From Latin ***mille*** = one thousand

millilitre a thousandth of a litre

mis-, miso-
denoting hating, hatred
combining form
From Greek *misos* = hate, hatred, from *misein* = to hate

misandry	hatred of men
misanthropic	hating people
misogyny	hatred of women

mon-, mono-
denoting one, single
combining form
From Greek *monos* = alone, only

monoclonal antibody	an antibody derived from a single cell clone
monocular	relating to one eye only
monorchid	having only one testicle
monozygotic twins	identical twins, developed from a single zygote

≈ Latin equivalent ▸ **uni-**

mons
a small rounded mass of fatty tissue on the body
noun
From Latin *mons*, genitive *montis* = mountain
Plural form **montes**

mons pubis	the mound of subcutaneous fatty tissue just above the genitals in humans

morbid
relating to or of the nature of disease
adjective
From Latin *morbidus* = sickly, diseased, from *morbus* = illness, disease

morbid anatomy	the study of diseased organs and tissues

morbidity
the ratio of incidence of an illness
noun
From Latin *morbidus* = sickly, diseased, from *morbus* = illness, disease

morbilli-
denoting measles
combining form
From medieval Latin *morbillus* = pustule, from Latin *morbus* = illness, disease

morph-, morpho-

| **morbilli**form | resembling measles |
| **morbilli**virus | a virus, different species of which are responsible for human measles, canine distemper, etc |

morph-, morpho-
denoting form, shape, structure
combining form
From Greek ***morphē*** = form, shape

| **morpho**genesis | the origin and development of a part, organ or organism |

-morphous
denoting a form, shape, structure of a specified type
combining form
From Greek ***morphē*** = form, shape

| iso**morphous** | similar in shape or structure |

muc-, muci-, muco-
denoting mucus; denoting mucous membrane
combining form
From Latin ***mucus*** = mucus

muciferous	secreting or conveying mucus
mucopurulent	relating to or consisting of mucus and pus
mucosanguineous	relating to or consisting of mucus and blood
mucoviscidosis	cystic fibrosis

mucosa
a mucous membrane
noun
From Latin ***mucosus*** = slimy, mucous, from ***mucus*** = mucus
Plural form **mucosae**
◆ Related words **mucosal** *adj* ▸relating to a mucous membrane

mucous
relating to, producing or resembling mucus
adjective
From Latin ***mucosus*** = slimy, mucous, from ***mucus*** = mucus

| **mucous** membrane | a lining of various tubular cavities of the body, eg the nose, with glands secreting mucus |

! Do not confuse with ▸**mucus**

mucus

the slimy fluid secreted by various membranes in the body, which it moistens and protects

noun

From Latin ***mucus*** = mucus

! Do not confuse with ▸**mucous**

multi-

denoting much, many

combining form

From Latin ***multus*** = much, many

multicellular	having or consisting of many cells
multifactorial	involving or caused by many different factors, especially a combination of genetic and environmental factors
multigravida	a pregnant woman who has had one or more previous pregnancies

≈ Greek equivalent ▸**poly-**

muscular

relating to a muscle or consisting of muscles

adjective

From modern Latin ***muscularis*** = muscular, from ***musculus*** = little mouse, muscle

muscular dystrophy	any of the forms of a hereditary disease in which muscles suffer progressive deterioration

musculo-

denoting muscle, muscular

combining form

From modern Latin ***muscularis*** = muscular, from ***musculus*** = little mouse, muscle

musculocutaneous	relating to or supplying the muscles and the skin
musculoskeletal	relating to the muscles and the skeleton

mut-, muta-

denoting mutation

combining form

From Latin ***mutare*** = to change

mutagen	a substance that causes mutations
muton	the smallest element of a gene capable of giving rise to a new form by mutation

mutant

a form resulting from mutation

noun

undergoing or resulting from mutation

adjective

From Latin ***mutans***, genitive ***mutantis*** = changing, from ***mutare*** = to change

myc-, mycet-, myceto-, myco-

denoting fungus

combining form

From Greek ***mykēs***, genitive ***mykētos*** = mushroom, fungus

mycetoma	Madura foot, a fungal disease of the foot and leg
mycosis	a disease due to the growth of a fungus
mycotoxicosis	poisoning caused by a poisonous substance produced by a fungus

! Do not confuse with ▸ **myx-, myxo-**

myel-, myelo-

denoting bone marrow; denoting the spinal cord

combining form

From Greek ***myelos*** = marrow

myelin	the substance forming the medullary sheath of nerve fibres
myelitis	inflammation of the spinal cord; inflammation of the bone marrow
myeloblast	an immature cell of bone marrow, found in the circulating blood only in diseased conditions
myeloma	a tumour of the bone marrow or composed of cells normally present in bone marrow

myeloid

relating to, resembling or of the nature of marrow; relating to the spinal cord

adjective

From Greek ***myelōdēs*** = like marrow, from ***myelos*** = marrow and ***-oeidēs*** = resembling, having the form of, from ***eidos*** = form, shape

my-, myo-

denoting muscle

combining form

From Greek ***mys***, genitive ***myos*** = muscle

myalgia	muscle pain
myasthenia	weakness of the muscles

| **myo**cardium | the muscular substance of the heart |
| **myo**tonic dystrophy | a muscle-wasting disease that causes muscle stiffness, weakness and wasting |

myopia
short-sightedness

noun

From Greek ***myōpia*** = short-sightedness, from ***myōps*** = short-sighted, from ***myein*** = to shut and ***ōps***, genitive ***ōpos*** = eye

◆ Related words **myopic** *adj* ▸short-sighted

myx-, myxo-
denoting mucus

combining form

From Greek ***myxa*** = mucus, slime

| **myx**oma | a tumour of jellylike or mucous substance that usually forms just beneath the skin |
| **myxo**virus | any of a group of related viruses causing influenza, mumps, etc |

! Do not confuse with ▸**myc-, mycet-, myeceto-, myco-**

Nn

naevus
a birthmark; a pigmented spot or an overgrowth of small blood vessels in the skin

noun

From Latin ***naevus*** = mole, wart, spot

Plural form **naevi**

nano-
denoting extremely small; denoting one billionth

combining form

From Latin ***nanus*** = dwarf, from Greek ***nanos*** = dwarf

| **nano**bot | a microscopically small robot |
| **nano**gram | one billionth of a gram |

narc-, narco-
denoting narcotic drugs; denoting numbness or torpor

combining form

From Greek ***narkē*** = numbness

narcolepsy	a condition marked by short attacks of irresistible drowsiness
narcosis	drowsiness, unconsciousness or other effects on the central nervous system produced by a narcotic
narcotherapy	the treatment of disturbed mental states by prolonged drug-induced sleep
narcotic	producing sleep, numbness and pain relief

naso-
denoting the nose
combining form
From Latin ***nasus*** = nose

nasofrontal	relating to the nose and the frontal bone
nasogastric tube	a tube passed into the stomach through the nose
nasopharynx	the part of the pharynx above the soft palate

≈ Greek equivalent ▸**rhin-, rhino-**

natal[1]
relating to or connected with birth
adjective
From Latin ***natalis*** = relating to or connected with birth, natal, from ***natus*** = born, from ***nasci*** = to be born

natal[2]
relating to the buttocks
adjective
From Latin ***natis*** = buttock
≈ Greek equivalent ▸**gluteal**

nates
the buttocks
noun
From Latin ***nates*** = buttocks, plural of ***natis*** = buttock
Singular form **natis**
◆ Related words **natiform** *adj* ▸resembling buttocks

natr-, natri-
denoting sodium
combining form
From new Latin ***natrium*** = sodium

| hyper**natr**aemia | an abnormally high level of sodium chloride in the blood, especially in infants |
| **natri**uresis | the excretion of sodium in the urine |

nausea

a feeling of sickness and inclination to vomit

noun

From Latin ***nausea***, from Greek ***nausia*** = seasickness, nausea, from Greek
naus = ship

necr-, necro-

denoting dead or a dead body

combining form

From Greek ***nekros*** (*adj*) = dead; (*n*) = dead body

necrophilia	a morbid, especially sexual attraction towards dead bodies
necropsy	a post-mortem examination
necrosis	the death of part of the living body
necrotomy	the dissection of a dead body; the surgical excision of necrosed bone from a living body

neo-

denoting new

combining form

From Greek ***neos*** = new, young

neocortex	the upper and most recently evolved part of the cerebral cortex, dealing with higher brain functions such as sight
neogenesis	the regeneration of tissue
neonate	a newly born child
neoplasm	a morbid new growth of tissue

nephr-, nephro-

denoting a kidney or kidneys

combining form

From Greek ***nephros*** = kidney

nephrectomy	the surgical removal of a kidney
nephritis	inflammation of the kidneys
nephrology	the study of the structure, functions and diseases of the kidneys

≈ Latin equivalent ▸ **ren-, reni-, reno-**

nerve

a cord consisting of bundles of fibres that conveys impulses of sensation or
movement between the brain or other centre and some part of the body

noun

From Latin ***nervus*** = sinew, tendon, nerve

◆ Related words **nervous** *adj* ▸ relating to the nerves

neur-, neuri-, neuro-

denoting a nerve, nerve cell, a nerve fibre, nerve tissue, or the nervous system (especially the brain and spinal cord)

combining form

From Greek **neuron** = sinew, tendon, nerve

neuralgia	paroxysmal intermittent pain along the course of a nerve
neurilemma	the external sheath of a nerve fibre
neuromuscular	relating to or affecting both nerves and muscles
neuroplasm	the protoplasm of a nerve cell
neurosurgery	surgery performed on the brain, spinal cord or other parts of the nervous system
neurotoxin	a substance poisonous to nerve tissue

neuron

a cell with the specialized function of transmitting nerve impulses, a nerve cell

noun

From Greek **neuron** = sinew, tendon, nerve

◆▸ Related words **neuronal** *or* **neuronic** *adj* ▸relating to a nerve cell

neutr-, neutro-

denoting neutral; denoting neutrophils

combining form

From Latin **neutralis** = neuter, from **neuter** = neither, neuter

neutropenia	an abnormally low number of neutrophils in the blood
neutrophil	a white blood cell with granular cytoplasm and a lobular nucleus; its cytoplasmic granules have no special affinity for acidic or basic stains but will stain slightly with either

noci-

denoting pain

combining form

From Latin **nocere** = to hurt, to harm

nociceptor	a pain receptor

noct-, nocti-

denoting night

combining form

From Latin **nox**, genitive **noctis** = night

noctambulism	sleepwalking
nocturia	urination during the night

≈ Greek equivalent ▸ **nyct-, nycto-**

node

a small lump or swelling consisting of tissue

noun

From Latin **nodus** = knot, knob, node

◆ Related words **nodal** *adj* ▸ relating to, consisting of or resembling a node or nodes

nos-, noso-

denoting disease

combining form

From Greek **nosos** = disease

nosography	the description of diseases
nosology	the study of diseases; the branch of medicine which deals with the classification of diseases
nosophobia	an abnormal fear of contracting a disease

-nosis

denoting disease

combining form

From Greek **nosos** = disease

Plural form **-noses**

zoo**nosis**	a disease of animals which can be transmitted to humans, such as rabies etc

nucle-, nucleo-

denoting a nucleus; denoting nucleic acid

combining form

From Latin **nucleus** = nut, kernel, from **nux**, genitive **nucis** = nut

nucleocapsid	the outer protein shell of a virus containing nucleic acid
nucleoplasm	the protoplasm in the nucleus of a cell

nuclear

relating to the nucleus of a cell; relating to, derived from, or powered by the fission or fusion of atomic nuclei

adjective

From Latin **nucleus** = nut, kernel, from **nux**, genitive **nucis** = nut

nuclear medicine	the diagnosis and treatment of disease using radiation detectors or radioactive materials
nuclear sexing	the testing of a person's sex by examining cells from inside the cheek which, in females, have a condensation of chromatin under the nuclear membrane

nucleus

a compartment within the interphase eukaryotic cell bounded by a double membrane and containing the genomic DNA (*biol*); a group of nerve cells in the central nervous system (*anat*)

noun

From Latin **nucleus** = nut, kernel, from **nux**, genitive **nucis** = nut

Plural form **nuclei**

null

having no significance

adjective

From Latin **nullus** = none, no

null hypothesis	the hypothesis that any difference between statistical populations has no significance

nulli-

denoting none, no

combining form

From Latin **nullus** = none, no

nullipara	a woman who has never given birth to a child, especially if she is not a virgin

nyct-, nycto-

denoting night or darkness

combining form

From Greek **nyx**, genitive **nyktos** = night

nyctalopia	night-blindness, abnormal difficulty in seeing in a faint light
nyctophobia	a pathological fear of the night or of darkness

≈ Latin equivalent ▸ **noct-, nocti-**

Oo

ob-, oc-, op-

denoting against, opposite

combining form

From Latin **ob** = towards, at, before, against

obstruent	causing obstruction in a passage in the body
occlusion	the bite or mode of meeting of the teeth
opposable thumb	the thumb of a primate, which can be placed with the front (ventral) surface opposite that of the fingers of the same hand

occipital

relating to the back of the head or skull

adjective

the occipital bone

noun

From medieval Latin **occipitalis**, from Latin **occiput**, genitive **occipitis** = the back of the head, from **ob** = against and **caput** = head

occipital bone	the bone at the back of the skull
occipital lobe	the posterior lobe in each cerebral hemisphere, dealing with the interpretation of vision

occiput

the back of the head or skull

noun

From Latin **occiput**, genitive **occipitis** = the back of the head, from **ob** = against and **caput** = head

Plural form **occipita** (or **occiputs**)

ocular

relating to the eye or to vision

adjective

From Latin **ocularis** = relating to the eyes, from **oculus** = eye

oculo-

denoting the eye or eyes

combining form

From Latin **oculus** = eye

oculomotor	relating to or causing movements of the eye

odont-, odonto-

denoting a tooth or teeth; denoting dentine

combining form

From Greek **odous**, genitive **odontos** = tooth

odontalgia	toothache
odontoblast	a dentine-forming cell
odontology	the study of the teeth

-odontia

denoting the teeth

combining form

From Greek **odous**, genitive **odontos** = tooth

hyp**odontia**	a condition in which someone has fewer teeth than normal
orth**odontia**	the rectification of crookedness in the teeth

-odynia

denoting pain in a specified part of the body

combining form

From Greek ***odynē*** = pain

gloss**odynia** pain in the tongue

oedema

a pathological accumulation of fluid in tissue spaces; dropsy

noun

From Greek ***oidēma***, genitive ***oidēmatos*** = swelling, tumour, from ***oidein*** = to swell, to become swollen

Plural form **oedemata** (or **oedemas**)

◆ Related words **oedematose** *or* **oedematous** *adj* ▸relating to oedema

oesophag-, oesophago-

denoting the gullet

combining form

From Greek ***oisophagos*** = gullet

oesophagitis inflammation of the oesophagus

oesophagoscope an instrument for viewing or treating the oesophagus

oesophagus

the gullet

noun

From Greek ***oisophagos*** = gullet

Plural form **oesophagi** (or **oesophaguses**)

◆ Related words **oesophageal** *adj* ▸relating to the gullet

-oid

denoting resembling or having the shape of something else (*adj*); denoting something that resembles or has the shape of something else (*n*)

combining form

From Greek ***-oeidēs*** = resembling, having the form of, from ***eidos*** = form, shape

aden**oid**s gland-like lymphoid tissue at the back of the nose

condyl**oid** resembling a ▸**condyle**

delt**oid** muscle the large triangular muscle of the shoulder

sial**oid** resembling saliva

trich**oid** hairlike

oleo-

denoting oil

combining form

From Latin ***oleum*** = oil

oleogranuloma   a granuloma resulting from an inflammatory reaction to deposits of oil

---

olig-, oligo-

denoting little, few

combining form

From Greek *oligos* = little, few

oligaemia   an abnormal deficiency of blood

oligocythaemia   a deficiency of red cells in the blood

oligospermia   the condition of having an abnormally low number of sperm cells in the semen, a major cause of male infertility

oliguria   a condition in which an abnormally low amount of urine is secreted in proportion to the liquid that has been drunk

---

-ology see ▸ -logy

-oma

denoting a tumour or abnormal growth

combining form

From Greek *-ōma* = an ending of nouns formed from verbs with an infinitive ending in *-oun*

Plural form **-omata** (or **-omas**)

angi**oma**   a tumour consisting of blood vessels

carcin**oma**   a cancer arising in epithelial tissue

---

omo-

denoting the shoulder or shoulder blade

combining form

From Greek *ōmos* = shoulder

omohyoid   relating to the shoulder blade and hyoid

omoplate   the shoulder blade or scapula

≈ Latin equivalent ▸ **scapul-, scapulo-**

---

omphal-, omphalo-

denoting the navel or umbilical cord

combining form

From Greek *omphalos* = navel, umbilical cord

omphalitis   inflammation of the navel

omphalocele   a hernia in which abdominal organs protrude into the navel

omphalotomy   the cutting of the umbilical cord

omphalic

relating to the navel or umbilical cord

adjective

From Greek **omphalikos**, from **omphalos** = navel, umbilical cord

≈ Latin equivalent ▸**umbilical**

omphalo- see ▸**omphal-, omphalo-**

onco-

denoting a tumour; denoting bulk or mass

combining form

From Greek **onkos** = bulk, mass, body

oncogene	a gene, which may be carried by a virus, that affects the normal metabolism of a cell in such a way that it becomes cancerous
oncogenesis	the formation of cancerous tumours
oncology	the study of tumours
oncometer	an instrument for measuring variations in the bulk of bodily organs

oneir-, oneiro-

denoting a dream or dreaming

combining form

From Greek **oneiros** = dream

oneirodynia	troubled sleep; a nightmare

onych-, onycho-

denoting the nails

combining form

From Greek **onyx**, genitive **onychos** = nail, talon, claw, hoof

onychitis	inflammation of the soft parts about the nail
onychocryptosis	ingrowing toenail

oo-

denoting egg, ovum

combining form

From Greek **ōion** = egg

oocyte	an ovum before it matures and begins to divide
oogenesis	the genesis and development of an ovum

≈ Latin equivalent ▸**ovi-, ovo-**

oophor-, oophoro-
denoting the ovary or ovaries
combining form
From Greek **ōiophoros** = egg-bearing, from **ōion** = egg and **phoros** = bearing, from **pherein** = to bear, to bring, to carry

| **oophor**ectomy | the removal of one or both ovaries, or of an ovarian tumour |
| **oophor**itis | inflammation of an ovary |

op- see ▸ ob-, oc-, op-

-opathic see ▸ -pathic

ophthalm-, ophthalmo-
denoting the eye
combining form
From Greek **ophthalmos** = eye

ophthalmitis	inflammation of the eye
ophthalmology	the study of the eye, its structure, functions and diseases
ophthalmoscope	a viewing instrument for examining the interior of the eye

ophthalmic
relating to the eye
adjective
From Greek **ophthalmikos** = relating to the eye, from **ophthalmos** = eye

ophthalmo- see ▸ ophthalm-, ophthalmo-

-opia
denoting a specified type of vision
combining form
From Greek **ōps**, genitive **ōpos** = eye

hypermetr**opia**	long-sightedness
my**opia**	short-sightedness
presby**opia**	difficulty in accommodating the eye to near vision, long-sightedness, a defect increasing with age

opisth-, opistho-
denoting behind, backwards
combining form
From Greek **opisthen** = behind, at the back

| **opistho**gnathous | having receding jaws |

opisthotonos   extreme arching backwards of the spine and neck as a result of spasm of the muscles in that region

≈ Latin equivalent ▸ **retro-**

-opsia
denoting a specified type of vision
combining form
From Greek *opsis* = sight, vision, seeing

chlor**opsia**	a disorder of the vision in which everything appears green
hemian**opsia**	blindness in half of the field of vision
heter**opsia**	different vision in each eye

-opsy
denoting examination
combining form
From Greek *opsis* = sight, vision, seeing

aut**opsy**	a post-mortem examination of a corpse
bi**opsy**	the surgical removal of tissue from a living body for diagnostic examination; a diagnostic examination of tissue surgically removed from a living body

---

oral
relating to the mouth; taken through the mouth; relating to the infant stage of development when satisfaction is obtained by sucking
adjective
From late Latin *oralis*, from Latin *os*, genitive *oris* = mouth

oral hygiene	the maintenance of healthy teeth and gums, as by careful cleaning, scaling, etc
oral rehydration therapy	the treatment of dehydration caused by diarrhoea etc with drinks of a water, glucose and salt solution

---

orch-, orchi-, orchid-
denoting a testicle
combining form
From Greek *orchis*, genitive *orchios* or *orcheōs* (not *orchidos*) = testicle

orchidectomy	the surgical removal of one or both testicles
orchitis	inflammation of one or both testicles

-orexia
denoting appetite
combining form

From Greek **orexis** = desire, appetite, from **oregein** = to stretch out, to desire

an**orexia**	a lack of appetite
orth**orexia**	an obsession with healthy eating

oro-

denoting the mouth

combining form

From Latin **os**, genitive **oris** = mouth

orofacial	relating to the mouth and face

orth-, ortho-

denoting straight, upright; denoting correct, right, normal

combining form

From Greek **orthos** = straight, upright, true, correct, real

orthodontic	relating to the rectification of crookedness in the teeth
orthognathous	having a normal lower jaw that neither protrudes nor recedes
orthopaedics	the branch of medicine concerned with the correction of disorders or deformities of the bones, joints, or muscles
orthoptics	the treatment and correction of defective eyesight by exercises and visual training
orthosis	a device that supports, corrects deformities in or improves the movement of the movable parts of the body

os[1]

a bone

noun

From Latin **os**, genitive **ossis** = bone

Plural form **ossa**

◆ Related words **osseous** *adj* ▸composed of or resembling bone; relating to or of the nature or structure of bone

os[2]

a mouth or mouthlike opening

noun

From Latin **os**, genitive **oris** = mouth

Plural form **ora**

osche-, oscheo-

denoting the scrotum

combining form

From Greek **oschē** = scrotum

oscheitis	inflammation of the scrotum
oscheoplasty	plastic surgery of the scrotum

oscheal

relating to the scrotum

adjective

From Greek ***osche*** = scrotum

-osis

denoting a condition or process; denoting a diseased condition

combining form

From Latin ***-osis***, from Greek ***-ōsis*** = an ending of nouns formed from verbs with an infinitive ending in ***-oun***

Plural form **-oses**

cirrh**osis**	a reaction of the liver to chronic damage characterized by regeneration of parenchyma, accompanied by fibrosis
dermat**osis**	a disease of the skin, especially one without inflammation
hidr**osis**	sweating, especially in excess
kyph**osis**	a hunchbacked condition
thromb**osis**	the formation of a thrombus (a blood clot within an intact vessel)

osm-, osmo-[1]

denoting smell, sense of smell

combining form

From Greek ***osmē*** = smell, sense of smell

osmatic	relating to or having a good sense of smell
osmic	relating to smells or to the sense of smell
osmidrosis	the secretion of sweat with an abnormally unpleasant smell

osm-, osmo-[2]

denoting diffusion

combining form

From Greek ***ōsmos*** = thrusting, pushing, from ***ōthein*** = to thrust, to push

osmoregulation	the process by which the body regulates the amount of water it contains and the concentration of various solutes and ions in its fluids

-osmia

denoting smell, sense of smell

combining form

From Greek ***osmē*** = smell, sense of smell

| anosmia | the partial or complete loss of the sense of smell |
| cacosmia | a disorder of the sense of smell in which someone constantly perceives unpleasant smells |

---

osmo- see ▶ osm-, osmo-

---

osmosis

the diffusion of a liquid through a semipermeable membrane
noun
From Greek **ōsmos** = thrusting, pushing, from **ōthein** = to thrust, to push

---

osmotic

relating to the diffusion of a liquid through a semipermeable membrane
adjective
From Greek **ōsmos** = thrusting, pushing, from **ōthein** = to thrust, to push

| **osmotic** pressure | the pressure exerted by a dissolved substance due to the motion of its molecules; a measure of this is the pressure that must be applied to a solution which is separated by a semipermeable membrane from a pure solvent in order to prevent the passage of the solvent through the membrane |

---

oste-, osteo-

denoting bone
combining form
From Greek **osteon** = bone

osteoarthritis	a form of arthritis in which the cartilages of the joint and the bone adjacent are worn away
osteochondrosis	a disease in which abnormal growth of cartilage or bone leads to degeneration of the cartilage, usually in the joints
osteogenesis	the formation of bone
osteoporosis	the development of a porous structure in bone as a result of loss of calcium, resulting in brittleness

---

-ostomy see ▶ -stomy

---

ot-, oto-

denoting the ear
combining form
From Greek **ous**, genitive **ōtos** = ear

| **ot**itis | inflammation of the ear |
| **oto**sclerosis | the formation of spongy bone in the capsule of the labyrinth of the ear and in the ossicles of the middle ear |

otoscope   a viewing instrument for examining the ear

≈ Latin equivalent ▸ **auri-**

---

otic
relating to the ear
adjective
From Greek **ōtikos** = relating to the ear, from **ous**, genitive **ōtos** = ear
≈ Latin equivalent ▸ **aural**

---

oto- see ▸ **ot-, oto-**

---

ovi-, ovo-
denoting egg, ovum
combining form
From Latin **ovum** = egg
   oviduct   the tube that conveys an egg from the ovary to the uterus

≈ Greek equivalent ▸ **oo-**

---

ovum
an egg cell or female gamete
noun
From Latin **ovum** = egg
Plural form **ova**

Pp

---

pachy-
denoting thick, especially abnormally thick; denoting the dura mater
combining form
From Greek **pachys** = thick
   pachydactyly   abnormal thickness of the fingers and toes
   pachymeningitis   meningitis of the dura mater of the brain and spinal cord

---

paed-, paedo-
denoting child, children
combining form
From Greek **pais**, genitive **paidos** = child
   paediatrics   the treatment of children's diseases
   paedodontics   the branch of dentistry concerned with the care of
                           children's teeth

palae-, palaeo-
denoting old
combining form
From Greek **palaios** = old

    palaeopathology   the pathological study of the ancient remains of animals and humans

    palaeothalamus   the part of the thalamus believed to have evolved earliest

palatal
relating to the palate
adjective
From Latin **palatum** = palate

palatine
relating to the palate
adjective
either of a pair of bones that form part of the roof of the mouth
noun
From Latin **palatum** = palate

palato-
denoting the palate
combining form
From Latin **palatum** = palate

    palatoglossal   relating to the palate and the tongue

    palatoplasty   plastic surgery of the palate

≈ Greek equivalent ▸**uran-, urano-**

palmar
relating to the palm of the hand
adjective
From Latin **palmaris** = a palm's length, a palm's width, from **palma** = palm

palpebral
relating to the eyelid
adjective
From Latin **palpebralis** = relating to or on the eyelids, from **palpebra** = eyelid

pan-, pant-, panto-
denoting all
combining form
From Greek **pas**, **pasa**, **pan**, genitive **pantos**, **pāsēs**, **pantos** = all

    panacea   a cure for all things

| **pan**demic | a disease that attacks great numbers of people in many different countries |
| **pan**ophthalmitis | inflammation of the whole eye |

par-, para-

denoting beside; denoting faulty, disordered, abnormal, false; denoting closely resembling or parallel to

combining form

From Greek ***para*** = from, beside, along, beyond

paraesthesia	an abnormal sensation in any part of the body
parainfluenza virus	any of a number of viruses causing influenza-like symptoms, especially in children
paralalia	a form of speech disturbance, particularly that in which a different sound or syllable is produced from the one intended
paramedic	a person who helps doctors or supplements medical work, especially a member of an ambulance crew
parathyroid	beside the thyroid
paratyphoid	a disease resembling typhoid

-para

denoting a woman who has given birth a specified number of times

combining form

From Latin ***parere*** = to bear

Plural form **-parae** (or **-paras**)

multi**para**	a woman who has given birth for the second or subsequent time, or is about to do so
nulli**para**	a woman who has never given birth to a child, especially if she is not a virgin
pluri**para**	a woman who has given birth for the second or subsequent time, or is about to do so

parasympathetic

adjective

relating to the parasympathetic nervous system, the part of the autonomic nervous system that promotes non-urgent physiological functions such as digestion and thus complements the sympathetic nervous system

From Greek ***para*** = beside and ***sympatheia*** = sympathy, from ***sympathēs*** = sympathetic, from ***syn*** = with and ***pathos*** = feeling, from ***paschein*** = to experience, to suffer

| **parasympathetic** nerve | a nerve of the parasympathetic nervous system |

paresis

a partial form of paralysis causing diminished activity of muscles but not diminishing sensation

noun

From Greek ***paresis*** = releasing, relaxing, from ***parienai*** = to let fall at the side, to relax

Plural form **pareses**

◆ Related words **paretic** *adj* ▸ relating to paresis

parietal

relating to or attached to the side or the inside of the wall of a cavity; relating to or near the parietal bone

adjective

a parietal bone

noun

From Latin ***parietalis*** = relating to walls, from ***paries***, genitive ***parietis*** = wall

parietal bone	either of the two bones which form part of the sides and top of the skull, between the frontal and the occipital
parietal cells	cells in the stomach lining that produce hydrochloric acid
parietal lobe	either of the divisions of the brain below the top of the skull

-parity

denoting the condition of having given birth a specified number of times

combining form

From Latin ***parere*** = to bear

multi**parity**	the condition of being a woman who has given birth for the second or subsequent time, or is about to do so
nulli**parity**	the condition of being a woman who has never given birth to a child, especially if she is not a virgin
primi**parity**	the condition of being a woman who has given birth for the first time only, or is about to do so

-parous

denoting giving birth

combining form

From Latin ***parere*** = to bear

multi**parous**	having given birth for the second or subsequent time, or about to do so
primi**parous**	having given birth for the first time only, or about to do so
vivi**parous**	producing living young that have already reached an advanced stage of development before delivery

-partum

denoting childbirth

combining form

From Latin ***partum***, accusative of ***partus*** = birth

ante**partum**	before childbirth
post**partum**	after childbirth

parv-, parvi-, parvo-

denoting small

combining form

From Latin ***parvus*** = small

parvovirus	any of a group of very small viruses which contain DNA and which are the causes of various diseases in mammals

path-, patho-

denoting disease, disorder

combining form

From Greek ***pathos*** = experience, misfortune, suffering, from ***paschein*** = to experience, to suffer

histo**patho**logy	the study of the effects of disease on the tissues of the body
pathogen	an organism or substance that causes disease
pathogenesis	the cause and development of a disease
pathologist	a person skilled in pathology; for example, anatomic pathologist – one who performs post-mortems, histopathologist – one who makes diagnoses from biopsy material, cytopathologist – one who makes diagnoses from examining cells derived from body fluids, aspirated through needles from tissues, or scraped from the surface of lesions
pathology	the study of diseases or abnormalities or, specifically, of the changes in tissues or organs that are associated with disease; a deviation from the healthy state

-pathic

denoting relating to or affected by a particular disease or disorder; denoting relating to treatment or therapy for a particular disease or disorder

combining form

From Greek ***pathikos*** = passive, from ***pathos*** = experience, misfortune, suffering, from ***paschein*** = to experience, to suffer

allo**pathic**	relating to the treatment of disease by inducing an effect that is different from the cause of the disease
neuro**pathic**	relating to or affected by nervous disease

patho- see ▸ path-, patho-

-pathy

denoting disease or disorder; denoting treatment or therapy for a particular disease or disorder

combining form

From Greek *-patheia*, from ***pathos*** = experience, misfortune, suffering, from ***paschein*** = to experience, to suffer

arthro**pathy**	a disease of the joints
cyano**pathy**	a disease characterized by bluish discoloration of the skin resulting from lack of oxygen in the blood
encephalo**pathy**	a degenerative brain disease
homeo**pathy**	a type of alternative medicine, based on the principle of treating diseases with small quantities of drugs that produce symptoms similar to those of the disease
myo**pathy**	a disease of the muscles or muscle tissue
osteo**pathy**	a system of healing or treatment consisting largely of manipulation of the bones and massage

pectoral

relating to for, on, or near the breast or chest

adjective

either of the two muscles situated on either side of the top half of the chest and responsible for certain arm and shoulder movements

noun

From Latin ***pectoralis*** = relating to the breast, pectoral, from ***pectus***, genitive ***pectoris*** = chest, breast, breastbone

pectoral girdle	the bony arch consisting of the shoulder-blade and collarbone

ped-, pedi-, pedo-

denoting the foot or feet

combining form

From Latin ***pes***, genitive ***pedis*** = foot

pedometer	an instrument for counting paces and so approximately measuring distance walked
peduncle	any stalk-like part in a body

≈ Greek equivalent ▶ **pod-, podo-**

pedal

relating to the foot or feet

adjective

From Latin ***pedalis*** = relating to the foot, from ***pes***, genitive ***pedis*** = foot

pedes see ▸ **pes**

pedi- see ▸ **ped-, pedi-, pedo-**

pedicle

a narrow stalk-like structure or short bony process

noun

From Latin **pediculus** = little foot, pedicle, from **pes**, genitive **pedis** = foot

pedo- see ▸ **ped-, pedi-, pedo-**

pellicle

a thin skin or film; a protein covering that preserves the shape of single-cell organisms

noun

From Latin **pellicula** = a small skin or hide, from **pellis** = skin

◆▸ Related words **pellicular** *adj* ▸relating to a pellicle

pelvic

relating to the bony cavity at the lower end of the trunk; relating to the cavity of the kidney

adjective

From Latin **pelvis** = basin

pelvic girdle *or* arch	the posterior bony arch with which the hind limbs articulate, consisting of the haunch bones (ilium, pubis and ischium united), which articulate with the sacrum
pelvic inflammatory disease	a damaging inflammatory condition affecting a woman's pelvic organs, especially the Fallopian tubes, caused by a bacterial infection

pelvis

the bony cavity at the lower end of the trunk, of which the part above the plane through the promontory of the sacrum and the pubic symphysis is the *false pelvis*, the part below the *true pelvis*; the bony frame enclosing it; the cavity of the kidney

noun

From Latin **pelvis** = basin

Plural form **pelves** (or **pelvises**)

renal **pelvis**	the cavity of the kidney

-penia

denoting deficiency, lack

combining form

From Greek *penia* = poverty, need, lack

neutro**penia**   an abnormally low number of neutrophils in the blood

thrombocyto**penia** an abnormal decrease in the number of platelets in the blood, causing haemorrhage

-penic

denoting relating to or characterized by a deficiency or lack of the specified thing

combining form

From Greek *penia* = poverty, need, lack

neutro**penic**   relating to or characterized by an abnormally low number of neutrophils in the blood

thrombocyto**penic** relating to or characterized by an abnormal decrease in the number of platelets in the blood, which causes haemorrhage

-pepsia

denoting digestion

combining form

From Greek *pepsis* = digestion, from *peptein* = to digest

dys**pepsia**   indigestion

eu**pepsia**   good digestion

peptic

relating to or promoting digestion; relating to pepsin or the digestive juices

adjective

From Greek *peptikos* = able to digest, promoting digestion, from *peptein* = to digest

peptic ulcer   an ulcer of the stomach, duodenum, etc

-peptic

denoting relating to, affected by, or caused by digestion of the specified kind

combining form

From Greek *peptikos* = able to digest, promoting digestion, from *peptein* = to digest

dys**peptic**   relating to, affected by, or arising from indigestion

eu**peptic**   relating to or having good digestion

peri-
denoting around, surrounding
combining form
From Greek ***peri*** = around

pericardium	the sac around the heart
perinatal	relating to the period around the birth of a baby, between the seventh month of pregnancy and the first month of the baby's life
periodontal	relating to tissues or regions around a tooth

≈ Latin equivalent ▸ **circum-**

pero-
denoting malformation
combining form
From Greek ***pēros*** = maimed

perodactyly	congenital malformation of the fingers or toes
peromelia	congenital malformation of the limbs

pes
the foot
noun
From Latin ***pes***, genitive ***pedis*** = foot
Plural form **pedes**

petr-, petro-
denoting hardness or density
combining form
From Greek ***petros*** = stone or ***petra*** = rock

osteo**petr**osis	a group of hereditary bone diseases in which bone becomes abnormally dense
petrosal	relating to the dense part of the temporal bone around the inner ear

-pexy
denoting fixation
combining form
From Greek ***pēxis*** = fixing, from ***pēgnunai*** = to fix

nephro**pexy**	the fixation of a floating kidney

! Do not confuse with ▸ **-plexy**

phac-, phaco-, phak-, phako-

denoting the lens of the eye

combining form

From Greek ***phakos*** = lentil

phacoemulsification	a surgical operation in which the lens of the eye is emulsified, before being removed and replaced by a plastic lens

phag-, phago-

denoting eating, consuming

combining form

From Greek ***phagein*** = to eat

phagedaena	hospital gangrene, rapidly spreading destructive ulceration, once common in hospitals
phagocyte	a white blood cell that engulfs bacteria and other harmful particles

-phagia

denoting the eating of the specified thing or in the specified way

combining form

From Greek ***phagein*** = to eat

aero**phagia**	the swallowing of air
copro**phagia**	the eating of faeces
dys**phagia**	difficulty in swallowing
hyalo**phagia**	a craving to eat glass

phago- see ▶ phag-, phago-

phak-, phako- see ▶ phac-, phaco-, phak-, phako-

phalanx

a bone of a finger or toe

noun

From Greek ***phalanx***, genitive ***phalangos*** = troop formation, bone of finger or toe

Plural form **phalanges**

phallic

relating to or resembling a phallus; relating to the stage of psychosexual development in which the child's interest and gratification is concentrated on his or her genital organs

adjective

From Greek ***phallikos*** = relating to the penis or a phallus, from ***phallos*** = penis, phallus

pharmac-, pharmaco-

denoting drugs or medicines

combining form

From Greek ***pharmakon*** = drug, medicine

pharmaceutical	relating to drugs or medicines or the science of preparing and dispensing them
pharmaco-dynamics	the science of the action of drugs on the body
pharmacokinetic	relating to the way the body deals with drugs
pharmacology	the study of drugs

pharyng-, pharyngo-

denoting the pharynx

combining form

From Greek ***pharynx***, genitive ***pharygos*** or ***pharyngos*** = throat

pharyngitis	inflammation of the mucous membrane of the pharynx
pharyngology	the study of the pharynx and its diseases
pharyngoscope	a viewing instrument for examining the pharynx
pharyngotomy	a surgical incision into the pharynx

pharynx

the cleft or cavity forming the upper part of the gullet, lying behind the nose, mouth, and larynx

noun

From Greek ***pharynx***, genitive ***pharyngos*** = throat

Plural form **pharynges** (or **pharynxes**)

◆ Related words **pharyngal** *or* **pharyngeal** *adj* ▸ relating to the pharynx

-pharynx

denoting a specified part of the pharynx

combining form

From Greek ***pharynx***, genitive ***pharyngos*** = throat

Plural form **-pharynges** (or **-pharynxes**)

naso**pharynx**	the part of the pharynx above the soft palate
oro**pharynx**	the part of the pharynx between the soft palate and the epiglottis

-phasia

denoting speech disorder

combining form

From Greek ***phanai*** = to say

a**phasia**	the inability to generate or understand speech

| dys**phasia** | difficulty in expressing or understanding thought in spoken or written words, caused by brain damage |

phen-, pheno-
denoting showing; denoting phenotype
combining form
From Greek ***phainein*** = to show

phenetics	a system of classification of organisms based on observable similarities and differences irrespective of whether or not the organisms are related
phenocopy	a copy of a genetic abnormality that is produced by the environment and cannot be inherited
phenotype	the observable characteristics of an organism produced by the interaction of genes and environment; a group of individuals having the same characteristics of this kind

-phil
denoting something that has an affinity for a specified thing
combining form
From Greek ***philos*** = loving, friend, from ***philein*** = to love, to like

acido**phil**	a cell that has an affinity for acid stains
baso**phil**	a white blood cell that has granules with an affinity for basic stains
neutro**phil**	a white blood cell with granular cytoplasm and a lobular nucleus; its cytoplasmic granules have no special affinity for acidic or basic stains but will stain slightly with either

-philia
denoting an abnormal fondness for or attraction to a specified type of person or a specified thing; denoting an excessive tendency towards a specified thing; denoting an affinity for a specified thing
combining form
From Greek ***philia*** = love, fondness, friendship, from ***philein*** = to love, to like

copro**philia**	an abnormal interest in faeces or defecation
haemo**philia**	a hereditary disease causing excessive bleeding when any blood vessel is even slightly injured
necro**philia**	a morbid, especially sexual attraction towards dead bodies

≈ Latin equivalent ▶ **-affin**

-philic
denoting being abnormally fond of or attracted to a specified type of person or a specified thing; denoting having an excessive tendency towards a

specified thing; denoting having an affinity for a specified thing
combining form
From Greek **philikos** = friendly, from **philein** = to love, to like

baso**philic**   having an affinity for basic stains

haemo**philic**   relating to, characterized by, or affected by excessive bleeding when any blood vessel is even slightly injured

necro**philic**   having a morbid, especially sexual attraction towards dead bodies

phleb-, phlebo-
denoting a vein
combining form
From Greek **phleps**, genitive **phlebos** = blood vessel, vein, artery

phlebitis   inflammation of the wall of a vein

phlebotomy   a surgical incision into a vein, or the extraction of blood from a vein using a hypodermic needle and syringe

≈ Latin equivalent ▸**vene-, veni-, veno-**

-phobia
denoting fear or hatred, especially a morbid or irrational one, of a specified thing
combining form
From Greek **phobos** = fear

agora**phobia**   a pathological fear of open spaces

arachno**phobia**   a pathological fear of spiders

claustro**phobia**   a pathological fear of confined spaces

emeto**phobia**   a pathological fear of vomiting

-phobic
denoting fearing or hating a specified thing, especially in a morbid or irrational way
combining form
From Greek **phobos** = fear

acro**phobic**   pathologically afraid of heights

hydro**phobic**   afraid of water (*psych*); repelling water (*biochem*)

phoco-
denoting abnormal shortness and closeness to the body
combining form
From Greek **phōkē** = seal

phocomelia   the condition of having one or more limbs like a seal's flippers, shortened and close to the body

phon-, phono-
denoting sound or voice
combining form
From Greek **phōnē** = sound, voice
phonasthenia weakness of the voice
phonocardiogram a visual record tracing of the sounds made by the heart

-phonia
denoting sound or voice
combining form
From Greek **phōnē** = sound, voice
a**phonia** loss of voice from hysteria, disease of the larynx or vocal cords, etc
dys**phonia** difficulty in producing voice sounds

-phonic
denoting speaking or producing sounds
combining form
From Greek **phōnikos** = vocal, from **phōnē** = sound, voice
dys**phonic** relating to, characterized by or experiencing difficulty in producing voice sounds

-phoria
denoting movement in the specified direction
combining form
From Greek **pherein** = to bear, to bring, to carry
eso**phoria** a tendency to squint inwards towards the nose
exo**phoria** a tendency to squint outwards away from the nose
hetero**phoria** a tendency to squint

-phoric
denoting moving in the specified direction
combining form
From Greek **pherein** = to bear, to bring, to carry
hetero**phoric** relating to, characterized by or having a tendency to squint

phot-, photo-
denoting light
combining form
From Greek **phōs**, **phōtos** = light
photalgia pain in the eyes due to bright light

photophobia	extreme sensitivity of the eyes to light (*pathol*); a pathological fear of or aversion to light (*psychol*)
photopsia	the appearance of flashes of light, owing to irritation of the retina
photoreceptor	a nerve-ending receiving light stimuli

phren-, phreno-
denoting the mind or brain; denoting the diaphragm
combining form
From Greek **phrēn**, genitive **phrenos** = midriff, heart, mind

phrenic nerve	the nerve that supplies the diaphragm
phrenitis	inflammation of the brain
phrenology	a would-be science of mental faculties supposed to be located in various parts of the skull and investigable by feeling the bumps on the outside of the head

-phrenia
denoting mental disorder of the specified type
combining form
From Greek **phrēn**, genitive **phrenos** = midriff, heart, mind

hebe**phrenia**	a form of insanity beginning in late childhood, arresting intellectual development, and ending in complete dementia
para**phrenia**	any mental disorder of the paranoid type
schizo**phrenia**	a psychosis marked by introversion, dissociation, inability to distinguish reality from unreality, delusions, etc

-phrenic
denoting relating to, characterized by or having a mental disorder of the specified type (*adj*); denoting someone who has the specified mental disorder (*n*)
combining form
From Greek **phrēn**, genitive **phrenos** = midriff, heart, mind

schizo**phrenic**	relating to, characterized by or having schizophrenia (*adj*); someone who has schizophrenia (*n*)

phys-, physio-
denoting nature; denoting physical
combining form
From Greek **physis** = growth, nature

physiology	the study of the processes of life in animals and plants
physiotherapy	the treatment of disease by remedies such as massage, fresh air, physical exercise, etc, rather than by drugs

-physis
denoting growth
combining form
From Greek **physis** = growth, nature
Plural form **-physes**

apo**physis**	an outgrowth from a bone
epi**physis**	any portion of a bone having its own centre of ossification
zygapo**physis**	any of the articulations of the vertebrae

pilo-
denoting hair
combining form
From Latin **pilus** = hair

pilomotor	causing hair to move
pilosebaceous	relating to hair follicles and sebaceous glands

pilus
a hair
noun
From Latin **pilus** = hair
Plural form **pili**

pimel-, pimelo-
denoting fat
combining form
From Greek **pimelē** = soft fat, lard

pimelopterygium	a wing-shaped area of thickened conjunctiva in the eye that contains fat

≈ Latin equivalent ▸ **adipo-**

piriform see ▸ -pyriform, piriform

pisiform
pea-shaped
adjective
a pea-shaped bone of the carpus
noun
From Latin **pisum** = pea and **forma** = shape

planta
the sole of the foot
noun

From Latin *planta* = sole

Plural form **plantae**

> **planta** pedis   the sole of the foot

◆ Related words **plantar** *adj* ▸relating to the sole of the foot

-plasia

denoting development, growth, formation
combining form

From modern Latin, from Greek *plasis* = moulding, from *plassein* = to form, to mould

achondro**plasia**	a hereditary disorder in which cartilage fails to convert to bone so that dwarfism results
dys**plasia**	abnormal development or growth of a cell, tissue, organ, etc
hetero**plasia**	the development of abnormal tissue or tissue in an abnormal place
hyper**plasia**	the overdevelopment of a part as a result of the excessive multiplication of its cells

-plasm

denoting a formative substance; denoting protoplasm
combining form

From Greek *plasma* = something formed or moulded, image, figure, from *plassein* = to form, to mould

cyto**plasm**	the protoplasm of a cell, which surrounds the nucleus
hyalo**plasm**	the clear fluid part of protoplasm
neo**plasm**	a morbid new growth of tissue
neuro**plasm**	the protoplasm of a nerve cell

plasma

the liquid part of blood, lymph, or milk
noun

From Greek *plasma* = something formed or moulded, image, figure, from *plassein* = to form, to mould

-plast

denoting a particle of living matter or an organized living cell
combining form

From Greek *plastos* = formed, moulded, from *plassein* = to form, to mould

bio**plast**	a minute portion of protoplasm
proto**plast**	the living part of a plant cell excluding the cell wall, or isolated from the cell wall by some means such as the action of enzymes

-plastic

denoting developing, growing, forming
combining form
From Greek ***plastikos*** = fit for moulding, plastic, from ***plassein*** = to form, to mould

hyper**plastic**	relating to the overdevelopment of a part as a result of the excessive multiplication of its cells
neo**plastic**	relating to the growth of morbid new tissue

-plasty

denoting plastic surgery involving a bodily part, tissue or a specified process
combining form
From Greek ***plastos*** = formed, moulded, from ***plassein*** = to form, to mould

angio**plasty**	a method of restoring a blocked or narrowed blood vessel to its original shape
facio**plasty**	reconstructive plastic surgery of the face
kerato**plasty**	the grafting of part of a healthy cornea to replace a piece made opaque by disease etc
mammo**plasty**	plastic surgery to change the shape of the breasts, as by the use of silicone implants etc
rhino**plasty**	plastic surgery of the nose

platy-

denoting broad, flat
combining form
From Greek ***platys*** = broad, flat

platycephalic	having the vault of the skull flattened
platysma	a broad sheet of muscle in the neck

pleo- or pleio-

denoting more or many
combining form
From Greek ***pleiōn*** or ***pleōn*** = more

pleocytosis	the presence of an abnormally large number of lymphocytes in the cerebrospinal fluid
pleomorphic	occuring in several forms

pleur-, pleuro-

denoting the pleura; denoting the side of the body
combining form
From Greek ***pleura*** = rib, side

pleurisy	inflammation of the pleura

pleurodynia	neuralgia of the muscles between the ribs
pleuropneumonia	pleurisy complicated with pneumonia
pleurotomy	a surgical incision into the pleura

pleura

a delicate serous membrane that covers the lung and lines the cavity of the chest

noun

From Greek ***pleura*** = rib, side

Plural form **pleurae**

| parietal **pleura** | the delicate serous membrane that lines the chest wall |
| visceral **pleura** | the delicate serous membrane that covers the lung |

pleural

relating to the delicate serous membrane that covers the lung and lines the chest wall

adjective

From Greek ***pleura*** = rib, side

| **pleural** cavity | the space between the pleura that covers the lung and the pleura that lines the chest wall |

pleuro see ▸ pleur-, pleuro-

plexus

a complex network of nerves, ganglia, blood vessels and lymphatic vessels anywhere in the body

noun

From Latin ***plexus*** = plaiting, from ***plectere*** = to plait, to braid, to interweave

Plural form **plexus** (or **plexuses**)

| choroid **plexus** | a vascular membrane projecting into the ventricles of the brain and secreting cerebrospinal fluid |
| solar **plexus** | a network of sympathetic nerves high in the back of the abdomen |

-plexy

denoting stroke

combining form

From Greek ***plēxis*** = stroke, percussion, from ***plēssein*** = to strike

| apo**plexy** | a sudden loss of sensation and motion, generally the result of haemorrhage or thrombosis in the brain |
| cata**plexy** | a condition of immobility induced by extreme emotion, eg shock |

! Do not confuse with ▸ **-pexy**

plica

a fold of tissue (*anat*); a matted condition of the hair (*pathol*)

noun

From medieval Latin **plica** = fold, from Latin **plicare** = to fold

Plural form **plicae** (or **plicas**)

◆ Related words **plicate** *adj* ▸having folds

plication

the folding and suturing of the walls of an organ to reduce its size

noun

From Latin **plicatus**, past participle of **plicare** = to fold

-plication

denoting the the folding and suturing of the walls of a specified organ to reduce its size

combining form

From Latin **plicatus**, past participle of **plicare** = to fold

fundo**plication**	a surgical operation in which the upper part of the stomach is folded together and sutured to the bottom part of the oesophagus as a treatment for gastro-oesophageal reflux disease

-ploid

denoting the possession of a specified number of chromosome sets

combining form

From Greek **plo-** = -fold and **-oeidēs** = resembling, having the form of, from **eidos** = form, shape

di**ploid**	having two sets of chromosomes, one set coming from each parent
eu**ploid**	having an even multiple of all the chromosomes in a set
ha**ploid**	having a single set of unpaired chromosomes
tri**ploid**	having three sets of chromosomes

pluri-

denoting more than two, several

combining form

From Latin **plus**, genitive **pluris** = more

pluripara	a woman who has given birth for the second or subsequent time, or is about to do so
pluripotent cell	a cell capable of developing into several different types of cell

pneum-, pneumat-, pneumato-, pneumo-

pneum-, pneumat-, pneumato-, pneumo-
denoting air, gas, breath, breathing
combining form
From Greek **pneuma**, genitive **pneumatos** = breath, breathing

pneumatometer	an instrument for measuring the quantity of air breathed or the force of breathing
pneumoperi-cardium	the presence of air in the pericardium

! Do not confuse with ▸ **pneum-, pneumo-, pneumon-, pneumono-**

pneum-, pneumo-, pneumon-, pneumono-
denoting the lung or lungs
combining form
From Greek **pneumōn**, genitive **pneumonos** = lung

pneumococcus	a bacterium in the respiratory tract which is a causative agent of pneumonia
pneumogastric	relating to the lungs and stomach
pneumonectomy	the surgical removal of lung tissue
pneumonia	inflammation of the lung (usually infective)
pneumonitis	inflammation of the lung (usually non-infective)

! Do not confuse with ▸ **pneum-, pneumat-, pneumato-, pneumo-**

≈ Latin equivalent ▸ **pulmo-, pulmon-, pulmono-**

-pnoea
denoting breathing
combining form
From Greek **pnoē** = breath, from **pnein** = to breathe

a**pnoea**	a cessation of breathing, especially a temporary one occurring in certain adults during sleep, or in newborn infants
dys**pnoea**	difficult or laboured breathing

-pnoeic
denoting breathing in the specified way
combining form
From Greek **pnoē** = breath, from **pnein** = to breathe

dys**pnoeic**	relating to, characterized by or experiencing difficult or laboured breathing

pod-, podo-
denoting the foot or the feet
combining form

From Greek **pous**, genitive **podos** = foot

podiatric	relating to the medical treatment of disorders of the foot
podology	the study of the feet

≈ Latin equivalent ▸ **ped-, pedi-, pedo-**

-poiesis

denoting production, formation

combining form

From Greek **poiēsis** = creation, production, from **poiein** = to make

erythro**poiesis**	the formation of red blood cells
haemato**poiesis**	the formation of blood
hidro**poiesis**	the production of sweat
leuco**poiesis**	the formation of white blood cells

---

poikilo-

denoting variegated, varied

combining form

From Greek **poikilos** = variegated, varied

poikilocyte	a red blood cell with an abnormal shape
poikiloderma	a condition in which the skin becomes mottled and atrophied
poikilothermic	having a variable blood-temperature, cold-blooded

---

pollex

the thumb

noun

From Latin **pollex**, genitive **pollicis** = thumb, big toe

Plural form **pollices**

◆ Related words **pollical** *adj* ▸relating to the thumb

---

poly-

denoting much, many, several, more than one; denoting affecting more than one part; denoting excessive

combining form

From Greek **polys**, **poleia**, **poly** = much, many

polyclonal	relating to or involving many clones
polycystic	containing many cysts
polycythaemia	an excess of red blood cells
polydactyly	a congenital condition in which someone has more than the normal number of fingers or toes
polydipsia	excessive thirst
polymyositis	inflammation of several muscles at the same time

polysomy   a condition in which one or more extra chromosomes, especially sex chromosomes, are present in the cells of the body

---

pompholyx

a vesicular eruption or eczema chiefly on the palms and soles
noun
From Greek **pompholyx**, genitive **pompholygos** = bubble, from **pomphos** = blister
◆ Related words **pompholygous** *adj* ▸relating to a pompholyx

---

pons

a connecting part
noun
From Latin **pons**, genitive **pontis** = bridge
Plural form **pontes**

    pons Varolii   a mass of fibres joining the hemispheres of the brain

◆ Related words **pontal, pontic, pontile** *or* **pontine** *adj* ▸relating to the pons of the brain

---

porta

a gate-like structure, especially the transverse fissure of the liver
noun
From Latin **porta** = gate
Plural form **portae** (or **portas**)

    porta hepatis   the transverse fissure of the liver

---

portal

relating to a gate-like structure; relating to the portal vein
adjective
From Latin **porta** = gate

    portal system   the portal vein with its tributaries etc
    portal vein   the vein that conveys to the liver the venous blood from the intestines, spleen, and stomach

---

post-

after, behind
combining form
From Latin **post** = behind, after

    post-mortem   after death (*adj, adv*); an autopsy (*n*)
    post-nasal drip   a condition in which mucus drips from the back of the nasal cavity into the throat, usually as a symptom of a cold or allergy

postnatal	relating to or typical of the period after birth
post-orbital	behind the eye or eye socket
post-operative	relating to the period just after a surgical operation
postpartum	after childbirth

◑ Opposite ▸ **ante-**

posterior

nearer to the back of the human body or to the back of a part of the human body

adjective

From Latin **posterior** = next, latter, later, posterior, comparative form of **posterus** = next, ensuing, future

◑ Opposite ▸ **anterior**

-praxia

denoting action

combining form

From Greek **praxis** = doing, action, from **prassein** = to do, to act

| a**praxia** | an inability, not due to paralysis, to perform voluntary purposeful movements of parts of the body, caused by brain lesion |
| dys**praxia** | an impaired ability to perform deliberate actions |

pre-

denoting before in time; denoting in front of; denoting the front part of

combining form

From Latin **prae** = before, in front of

precancerous	showing structural alterations recognized as associated with the subsequent development of cancer
precordial	in front of the heart
premandibular	in front of the lower jaw
premolar	in front of the true molar teeth
prenatal	before birth
presternum	the front part of the sternum

prim-, primi-

denoting first

combining form

From Latin **primus** = first

| **primi**gravida | a woman who is pregnant for the first time |
| **primi**para | a woman who has given birth for the first time only, or is about to do so |

primordial   relating to an early stage in growth

≈ Greek equivalent ▸ **prot-, proto-**

primary
first in order
adjective
From Latin ***primarius*** = first, chief, principal

primary care   the first level of health care, as provided by a general practitioner or nurse

primi- see ▸ **prim-, primi-**

pro-[1]
denoting forward; denoting in favour of, supporting, backing
combining form
From Latin ***pro*** = before, in front of, on behalf of, in favour of

pro-choice   upholding or supporting the right of a woman to have an abortion

prolapse   a falling down or out of place of an organ or tissue, especially the womb

pro-life   opposing abortion, euthanasia and experimentation on human embryos

pro-[2]
denoting before in time or place; denoting earlier than; denoting in front of; denoting the front part of; denoting primitive or rudimentary
combining form
From Greek ***pro*** = before, in front of

progeria   a rare disease causing premature ageing in children

prognathism   a condition in which one jaw projects farther than the other

prognosis   a forecast of the course of a disease

pronephros   the front portion of the kidney, functional in the embryo but functionless and often absent in the adult

prophase   the first stage of mitosis or meiosis during which chromosomes condense and become recognizably discrete

prophylaxis   preventive treatment against diseases etc

proct-, procto-
denoting the rectum or anus
combining form

From Greek **prōktos** = anus

proctalgia	neuralgic pain in the rectum
proctitis	inflammation of the rectum
proctology	the study and treatment of the anus and rectum
proctoscope	a viewing instrument for examining the rectum

≈ Latin equivalent ‣ **ano-; recto-**

---

prone

lying face downwards; with the palm of the hand facing downwards
adjective
From Latin **pronus** = bent forwards
◑ Opposite ‣ **supine**

---

proprio-

denoting one's own, self
combining form
From Latin **proprius** = own

proprioreceptor	a sensory nerve ending that receives stimuli signalling the relative positions of body parts

---

prosop-, prosopo-

denoting the face
combining form
From Greek **prosōpon** = face

prosopagnosia	the inability to recognize faces of familiar people
prosopodynia	facial pain

---

prot-, proto-

denoting first; denoting primitive
combining form
From Greek **prōtos** = first

protanopia	a form of colour blindness in which red and green are confused because the retina does not respond to red, the first primary colour
protopathic	relating to a certain type of nerve which is only affected by the coarser stimuli, eg pain; relating to this kind of reaction

≈ Latin equivalent ‣ **prim-, primi-**

---

proximal

nearest to the point of attachment
adjective

From Latin **proximus** = nearest, next
◑ Opposite ▸**distal**

pseud-, pseudo-
denoting false
combining form
From Greek **pseudēs** = false

pseudaesthesia	imaginary feeling, eg in an amputated limb
pseudocyesis	phantom pregnancy
pseudoherm-aphroditism	a congenital condition in which a man has external genitalia resembling those of a woman, and vice versa

pter-, ptero-
denoting feather, wing
combining form
From Greek **pteron** = feather, wing

pterion	the suture where the frontal, squamosal and parietal bones meet the wing of the sphenoid

-ptosis
denoting falling, downward displacement, prolapse
combining form
From Greek **ptōsis** = falling, fall, from **piptein** = to fall
Plural form **-ptoses**

apo**ptosis**	the controlled destruction ('falling away') of cells in a living organism
nephro**ptosis**	floating kidney
pro**ptosis**	forward displacement, especially of the eye

-ptotic
denoting falling, being displaced downwards, suffering prolapse
combining form
From Greek **ptōtikos**, from **piptein** = to fall

apo**ptotic**	relating to the controlled destruction of cells in a living organism

ptyal-, ptyalo-
denoting saliva
combining form
From Greek **ptyalon** = sputum, saliva, from **ptyein** = to spit

ptyalagogue	anything that stimulates a flow of saliva
ptyalism	an excessive flow of saliva
ptyalorrhoea	the excessive secretion of saliva

puerperal

relating to childbirth

adjective

From Latin ***puerpera*** = woman in labour, from ***puer*** = child and ***parere*** = to bear

puerperal fever	formerly any fever occurring in connection with childbirth; now confined to endometritis or septicaemia caused by the introduction of bacteria into the genital tract
puerperal psychosis	a mental illness sometimes occurring after childbirth

pulmo-, pulmon-, pulmono-

denoting the lung; denoting the pulmonary artery

combining form

From Latin ***pulmo***, genitive ***pulomonis*** = lung

pulmoaortic	relating to the pulmonary artery and the aorta
pulmonic	relating to the lungs
pulmonology	the study of the lungs and the respiratory system

≈ Greek equivalent ▸ **pneum-, pneumo-, pneumon-, pneumono-**

pulmonary

relating to the lungs or respiratory cavity; leading to or from the lungs; diseased or weak in the lungs

adjective

From Latin ***pulmonarius*** = diseased in the lungs, consumptive, good for the lungs, from ***pulmo***, genitive ***pulomonis*** = lung

pulmonary artery	the artery that brings blood from the heart to the lungs
pulmonary embolism	the presence of one or more obstructing emboli (masses that obstruct the circulation), usually thrombotic, in the pulmonary artery

pulmono see ▸ pulmo-, pulmon-, pulmono-

py-, pyo-

denoting pus

combining form

From Greek ***pyon*** = pus

em**py**ema	a collection of pus in any cavity, especially the pleura
pyaemia	infection of the blood with bacteria from a septic focus, with abscesses in different parts of the body
pyoderma	a skin infection in which pus is formed
pyogenesis	the formation of pus

pyel-, pyelo-
denoting the pelvis of the kidney
combining form
From Greek **pyelos** = trough

pyelitis	inflammation of the pelvis of the kidney
pyelogram	an X-ray picture of the pelvis of the kidney, the kidney and the ureter
pyelonephritis	inflammation of the kidney and the pelvis of the kidney

! Do not confuse with ▸ **pyl-, pyle-**

pyg-, pygo-
denoting the buttocks
combining form
From Greek **pygē** = buttocks

pygalgia	pain in the buttocks

pykn-, pykno-
denoting dense, thick
combining form
From Greek **pyknos** = close, compact, dense

pyknic	characterized by short squat stature, small hands and feet, relatively short limbs, domed abdomen, short neck, and round face
pyknodysostosis	a rare inherited bone disease characterized by short stature and fragility and thickening of the bones
pyknosis	the shrinkage of the stainable material of a nucleus into a deeply staining mass, usually a feature of cell degeneration

pyl-, pyle-
denoting the portal vein
combining form
From Greek **pylē** = gate, door, entrance, portal vein

pylephlebitis	inflammation of the portal vein
pylethrombosis	thrombosis of the portal vein

! Do not confuse with ▸ **pyel-, pyelo-**

pylor-, pyloro-
denoting the pylorus
combining form
From Greek **pylōros** = gate-keeper, pylorus, from **pylē** = gate and **ouros** = guardian

| **pylor**ectomy | the surgical removal of all or part of the pylorus |
| **pyloro**duodenal | relating to the pylorus and the duodenum |

pylorus

the opening from the stomach to the intestines

noun

From Greek **pylōros** = gate-keeper, pylorus, from **pylē** = gate and
ouros = guardian

Plural form **pylori**

◆ Related words **pyloric** *adj* ▸relating to the opening from the stomach to the
intestines

---

pyo- see ▸ **py-, pyo-**

---

pyr-, pyro-

denoting fire, heat, burning sensation, fever

combining form

From Greek **pyr**, genitive **pyros** = fire, fever

pyrogen	a substance causing heat or fever
pyromania	an obsessive urge to set fire to things
pyrosis	heartburn

---

pyret-, pyreto-

denoting fever

combining form

From Greek **pyretos** = burning heat, fever, from **pyr**, genitive **pyros** = fire, fever

| **pyret**ic | relating to, of the nature of or for the cure of fever |
| **pyreto**logy | the study of fevers |

---

pyrexia

fever

noun

From modern Latin, from Greek **pyressein** = to be feverish, from **pyr**, genitive
pyros = fire, fever

◆ Related words **pyrexic** *adj* ▸relating to fever

---

pyriform, piriform

pear-shaped

adjective

From modern Latin **pyriformis**, from **pyrum**, a misspelling of Latin **pirum** = pear
and Latin **forma** = shape

---

pyro- see ▸ **pyr-, pyro-**

Qq

quadr-, quadri-
　denoting four
　combining form
　From Latin **quadr-**, **quadri-**, from **quattuor** = four

quadratus	a four-sided muscle
quadriceps	the large four-part muscle that runs down the front of the thigh and extends the leg
quadriplegia	paralysis of all four limbs

　≈ Greek equivalent ▸ **tetr-, tetra-**

Rr

rachi-, rachio-
　denoting the spine
　combining form
　From Greek **rhachis** = lower back, spine, backbone

rachischisis	a severe form of spina bifida
rachiotomy	a surgical incision into the backbone to obtain access to the spinal cord

radius
　the outer bone of the forearm in a supine position
　noun
　From Latin **radius** = rod, spoke, ray, radius
　Plural form **radii** (or **radiuses**)
　◆ Related words **radial** *adj* ▸ relating to or near the radius

radix
　a root
　noun
　From Latin **radix**, genitive **radicis** = root
　Plural form **radices**

ramus
　a branch of anything, especially a nerve; a process of a bone; the mandible or its ascending part
　noun

From Latin **ramus** = branch
Plural form **rami**

raphe
a seam or ridge in an organ or tissue, usually marking where two halves meet, especially that between the halves of the brain
noun
From modern Latin, from Greek **rhaphē** = seam, suture, stitching, sewing, from **rhaptein** = to sew
Plural form **raphae**

rect-, recto-
denoting the rectum
combining form
From Latin **(intestinum) rectum** = straight (intestine), from **rectus** = straight, right

rectitis   inflammation of the rectum
rectocele   a hernia of the rectum into the vagina

≈Greek equivalent ▸**proct-, procto-**

rectum
the terminal part of the large intestine
noun
From Latin **(intestinum) rectum** = straight (intestine), from **rectus** = straight, right
Plural form **recta** (or **rectums**)
◆ Related words **rectal** *adj* ▸relating to the rectum

rectus
a straight muscle
noun
From Latin **rectus** = straight, right
Plural form **recti**

remedial
tending or intended to cure a disease; relating to the teaching of children with learning difficulties
adjective
From Latin **remedialis** = healing, remedial, from **remedium** = cure, remedy

ren-, reni-, reno-
denoting the kidneys
combining form
From Latin **renes** = kidneys

renin   a protein enzyme secreted by the kidneys into the bloodstream, where it helps to maintain the blood pressure

renography   radiography of the kidneys

≈ Greek equivalent ▸ **nephr-, nephro-**

-renal

denoting the kidneys

combining form

From Latin **renalis** = relating to the kidneys, renal, from **renes** = kidneys

ad**renal**   next to the kidneys

supra**renal**   above the kidneys

reni-, reno- see ▸ ren-, reni-, reno-

rete

a network, eg of blood vessels or nerves

noun

From Latin **rete**, genitive **retis** = net

Plural form **retia**

◆ Related words **retial** *adj* ▸ relating to a network, eg of blood vessels or nerves

reticulo-

denoting a network

combining form

From Latin **reticulum** = little net

reticulocyte   an immature red blood cell that exhibits a reticulated appearance when stained

reticulo-   the network of phagocytic cells extending throughout
endothelial   lymphoid and other organs which is involved in the
system   uptake and clearance of foreign particles from the blood

reticulum

a network, eg of cells, fibres, tubules or blood vessels

noun

From Latin **reticulum** = little net

Plural form **reticula**

◆ Related words **reticular** *adj* ▸ relating to a network, eg of cells, fibres, tubules or blood vessels

retro-

denoting back, backwards; denoting behind

combining form

From Latin **retro** = backwards, behind

retrobulbar	behind the eyeball
retroflexion	the bending back of an organ
retrolental	behind the lens of the eye
retropulsion	a tendency to walk backwards experienced by some people with Parkinson's disease

≈ Greek equivalent ▸**opisth-, opistho-**

rhin-, rhino-
denoting the nose
combining form
From Greek **rhis**, genitive **rhinos** = nose

rhinencephalon	the olfactory lobe of the brain
rhinitis	inflammation of the mucous membrane of the nose
rhinoplasty	plastic surgery of the nose
rhinorrhagia	excessive nose-bleeding

≈ Latin equivalent ▸**naso-**

rhiz-, rhizo-
denoting a root or roots
combining form
From Greek **rhiza** = root

rhizonychia	the root of a nail
rhizotomy	a surgical operation in which the roots of spinal nerves are cut, usually to relieve pain

rigor
a sense of chilliness with shivering and contraction of the erector pili muscles of the skin, a preliminary symptom of many bacterial diseases; stiffness or rigidity
noun
From Latin **rigor** = stiffness, chilliness

rigor mortis	the stiffening of the body after death

rostr-, rostri-, rostro-
denoting a part resembling a beak; denoting the front part of the body, especially the nose or mouth
combining form
From Latin **rostrum** = beak, snout, muzzle

rostriform	beak-shaped
rostro-inferior	relating to the front and lower part of an organ or body part

rostrum

a part resembling a beak

noun

From Latin ***rostrum*** = beak, snout, muzzle

Plural form **rostra** (or **rostrums**)

◆ Related words **rostral** *adj* ▸resembling a beak; relating to or near the upper or head end of the body, especially the nose or mouth

-rrhage

denoting an abnormal discharge

combining form

From Greek ***-rrhagia*** = bursting, from ***rhēgnynai*** = to break, to burst

haemo**rrhage**	a discharge of blood from the blood vessels

-rrhagia

denoting an abnormal or excessive discharge

combining form

From Greek ***-rrhagia*** = bursting, from ***rhēgnynai*** = to break, to burst

meno**rrhagia**	an excessive flow of blood during menstruation
metro**rrhagia**	bleeding from the uterus between menstrual periods

-rrhaphy

denoting suturing

combining form

From Greek ***rhaphē*** = seam, suture, stitching, sewing, from ***rhaptein*** = to sew, to stitch

hernio**rrhaphy**	the surgical repair of a hernia by an operation involving suturing
teno**rrhaphy**	the surgical repair of a split or torn tendon by an operation involving suturing

-rrhexis

denoting rupture

combining form

From Greek ***rrhēxis*** = breaking, bursting, from ***rhēgnynai*** = to break, to burst

arterio**rrhexis**	the rupture of an artery
hepato**rrhexis**	the rupture of the liver
metro**rrhexis**	the rupture of the uterus
phlebo**rrhexis**	the rupture of a vein

-rrhoea

denoting a flow or discharge

combining form

From Greek **rhoia** = flow, flux, from **rhein** = to flow

blenno**rrhoea**	discharge of mucus
dia**rrhoea**	a condition in which faeces are either more frequent or more liquid than usual
dysmeno**rrhoea**	difficult or painful menstruation
leuco**rrhoea**	an abnormal discharge of whitish mucus or mucus and pus from the vagina
logo**rrhoea**	uncontrolled or incoherent talkativeness

---

ruga

a crease or fold in an organ or body part

noun

From Latin **ruga** = wrinkle, crease, fold

Plural form **rugae**

◆ Related words **rugose** *or* **rugate** *adj* ▸having creases or folds

Ss

---

sacchar-, sacchari-, saccharo-

denoting sugar

combining form

From Latin **saccharum**, from Greek **sakcharon** = sugar

saccharify	to convert or break down starch into sugar or sugars
Saccharomyces	the yeast genus of ascomycete fungi, members of which ferment sugars

---

saccus

a sac or pouch

noun

From Latin **saccus** = sack, bag

Plural form **sacci**

---

sacr-, sacro-

denoting the sacrum

combining form

From Latin **(os) sacrum** = holy (bone)

sacralgia	pain in the sacrum or in the region of the sacrum
sacrococcygeal	relating to the sacrum and the coccyx
sacroiliac	relating to the articulation of the sacrum and ilium (*adj*); the sacroiliac joint (*n*)

sacrum

a triangular bone composed of five fused vertebrae wedged between the two innominate bones, so as to form the keystone of the pelvic arch

noun

From Latin *(os) sacrum* = holy (bone)

Plural form **sacra** (or **sacrums**)

◑ Related words **sacral** *adj* ▸relating to the sacrum

sagittal

relating or parallel to the sagittal suture

adjective

From Latin *sagitta* = arrow

sagittal plane	the plane that runs down the centre of the body from the sagittal suture, dividing the body into left and right halves
sagittal suture	the serrated join between the two parietal bones that form the top and sides of the skull

salping-, salpingo-

denoting a Fallopian tube; denoting a Eustachian tube

combining form

From Greek *salpinx*, genitive *salpingos* = trumpet

salpingectomy	the surgical removal of a Fallopian tube
salpingitis	inflammation of a tube, especially one or both Fallopian tubes

≈ Latin equivalent ▸**tub-, tubo-**

salpinx

either of the Fallopian tubes, leading from the ovary to the uterus; the Eustachian tube, leading from the middle ear to the pharynx

noun

From Greek *salpinx*, genitive *salpingos* = trumpet

Plural form **salpinges**

sanative

healing

adjective

From Latin *sanare* = to heal

sangui-, sanguin-, sanguino-

denoting blood

combining form

From Latin *sanguis*, genitive *sanguinis* = blood

con**sanguin**ity   relationship by blood as opposed to affinity or relationship by marriage

muco**sanguin**eous   relating to or consisting of mucus and blood

sanguiferous   conveying blood

≈ Greek equivalent ▸ **haem-, haemat-, haemato-, haemo-**

sapr-, sapro-

denoting rotten or decaying matter; denoting putrefaction

combining form

From Greek **sapros** = rotten, putrid

sapraemia   blood poisoning resulting from the presence of toxins of saprophytic bacteria in the blood

saprophyte   a fungus or bacterium that feeds upon dead and decaying organic matter

sarc-, sarco-

denoting flesh or fleshy tissue; denoting muscle

combining form

From Greek **sarx**, genitive **sarkos** = flesh

sarcolemma   the cell membrane enclosing a muscle fibre

sarcomere   a unit of myofibril in muscle

sarcoplasm   the protoplasmic substance separating the fibrils in muscle fibres

sartorius

a narrow ribbon-like muscle at the front of the thigh, the longest muscle in the body, helping to flex the knee

noun

From modern Latin **(musculus) sartorius** = tailor's (muscle), from Latin **sartor** = patcher, mender, from **sarcire** = to patch, to mend. The muscle is stretched when one sits in the cross-legged position traditionally adopted by tailors while sewing

Plural form **sartorii**

◆▸ Related words **sartorial** *adj* ▸ relating to the sartorius

scaph-, scapho-

denoting boat-shaped

combining form

From Greek **skaphē** = light boat, skiff

scaphocephaly   abnormal length and narrowness of the head

scaphoid bone   a boat-shaped bone of the wrist or ankle joint, the navicular bone

scapul-, scapulo-

denoting a shoulder blade or shoulder blades

combining form

From Latin *scapula* = shoulder blade, shoulder

scapuloclavicular   relating to the shoulder blade and the collarbone

scapulohumeral   relating to the shoulder blade and the bone of the upper arm

≈ Greek equivalent ▸**omo-**

scapula

a shoulder blade

noun

From Latin *scapula* = shoulder blade, shoulder

Plural form **scapulae** (or **scapulas**)

◆ Related words **scapular** *adj* ▸relating to the shoulder blade or shoulder

scapulo- see ▸ scapul-, scapulo-

-schisis

denoting cleaving or splitting

combining form

From Greek *schisis* = splitting, cleaving, parting, from *schizein* = to split, to cleave to part

rachi**schisis**   a severe form of spina bifida

retino**schisis**   the splitting of the retina

schist-, schisto-

denoting a split

combining form

From Greek *schistos* = split, cloven, divided, from *schizein* = to split, to cleave

schistocyte   a fragmenting red blood cell; a fragment of a red blood cell

schistoglossia   a condition in which the tongue is fissured

schiz-, schizo-

denoting a split, cleft or division; denoting schizophrenia

combining form

From Greek *schizein* = to split, to cleave

schizo-affective   marked by symptoms of schizophrenia and manic-depressiveness

schizogony   reproduction in protozoans by multiple fission of the nucleus followed by segmentation of the cytoplasm

| **schiz**oid | showing qualities of a schizophrenic personality, such as asocial behaviour, introversion, tendency to fantasy, but without definite mental disorder |
| **schizo**phrenia | a psychosis marked by introversion, dissociation, inability to distinguish reality from unreality, delusions, etc |

scler-, sclero-

denoting hard; denoting the sclera
combining form
From Greek ***skleros*** = hard

scleroderma	hardness and contraction of the body's connective tissue in which the skin becomes thickened by substitution of fibrous tissue for subcutaneous fat
scleroma	morbid hardening; a hardened area of mucous membrane or skin, eg forming nodules in the nose
sclerosis	morbid hardening, eg of arteries by deposition of fatty plaques
sclerotomy	a surgical incision into the sclera

scoli-, scolio-

denoting crooked
combining form
From Greek ***skolios*** = curved, bent, bent sideways

kypho**scoli**osis	a condition in which the spine is abnormally bent forwards and to the side
scoliosis	abnormal sideways curvature of the spine
scoliorachitic	affected by abnormal sideways curvature of the spine and rickets

-scope

denoting an instrument for viewing, examining, or detecting something
combining form
From modern Latin ***-scopium***, from Greek ***skopein*** = to look at

auri**scope**	a viewing instrument for examining the ear
coelo**scope**	a viewing instrument for examining the interior of a body cavity
colpo**scope**	a viewing instrument for examining the vagina and cervix
endo**scope**	a viewing instrument for examining the cavities of internal organs
micro**scope**	an instrument for viewing very small objects
ophthalmo**scope**	a viewing instrument for examining the interior of the eye
procto**scope**	a viewing instrument for examining the rectum

-scopy

denoting viewing, examining, or observing

combining form

From Greek **skopia** = watch, from **skopein** = to look at

amnio**scopy**	an examination of the interior of the amnion with a viewing instrument
coelio**scopy**	an examination of interior of the abdomen with a viewing instrument
endo**scopy**	any technique for viewing internal organs, such as by fibre-optic apparatus
laparo**scopy**	a surgical examination by means of a tube-shaped optical instrument which permits examination of the internal organs from outside, also used in female sterilization procedures

scot-, scoto-

denoting dark, darkness

combining form

From Greek **skotos** = darkness

scotoma	an area of abnormal or absent vision within the visual field, a blind spot due to disease of the retina or optic nerve
scotometer	an instrument for identifying defects in the visual field
scotopia	vision in dim light

seb-, sebi-, sebo-

denoting sebum

combining form

From Latin **sebum** = tallow, suet, grease

sebiferous	bearing fatty matter
seborrhoea	an excessive discharge of sebum from the sebaceous glands

sebaceous

relating to, resembling, of the nature of or secreting sebum

adjective

From Latin **sebaceus** = tallow candle, from **sebum** = tallow, suet, grease

sebaceous cyst	a cyst arising in a sebaceous gland
sebaceous gland	a gland in the skin that secretes sebum

! Do not confuse with ▸ **setaceous**

sebum

the fatty secretion that lubricates the hair and skin

noun

From Latin **sebum** = tallow, suet, grease

semi-

denoting half; denoting nearly, partly, incompletely

combining form

From Latin **semi-** = half-

semicoma	an unconscious state approaching coma
semilunar valve	either of the half-moon-shaped valves of the aorta and pulmonary artery that prevent regurgitation of blood into the heart

≈ Greek equivalent ▸**hemi-**

semin-, semini-, semino-

denoting semen

combining form

From Latin **semen**, genitive **seminis** seed, semen

semeniferous	producing or conveying semen
seminology	the study of semen and spermatozoa
seminoma	a malignant tumour of the testicle

seminal

relating to or containing semen

adjective

From Latin **seminalis** = relating to seed or semen, seminal, from **semen**, genitive **seminis** seed, semen

seminal fluid	semen
seminal vesicle	either of a pair of glands that secrete the fluid component of semen and open into the vas deferens

semini-, semino- see ▸semin-, semini-, semino-

sepsis

putrefaction; invasion by pathogenic bacteria

noun

From Greek **sēpsis** = putrefaction, decay, from **sēpein** = to make rotten or putrid

Plural form **sepses**

◆ Related words **septic** *adj* ▸affected by bacteria from a diseased wound, putrefying; caused by bacteria from a diseased wound

sept-, septi-, septem-
denoting seven
combining form
From Latin **septem** = seven

septigravida   a woman who is pregnant for the seventh time

! Do not confuse with ▸ **sept-, septi-, septo-**; **sept-, septo-**; **septic-, septico-**

sept-, septi-, septo-
denoting sepsis
combining form
From Greek **sēptos** = putrefactive, from **sēpein** = to make rotten or putrid

septimetritis   inflammation of the uterus due to sepsis

! Do not confuse with ▸ **sept-, septi-, septem-**; **sept-, septo-**; **septic-, septico-**

sept-, septo-
denoting a septum, especially the nasal septum
combining form
From Latin **saeptum** = fence, wall, enclosure, from **saepire** = to enclose

septectomy   the surgical removal of a septum, especially the nasal septum

septoplasty   plastic surgery of the nasal septum

! Do not confuse with ▸ **sept-, septi-, septem-**; **sept-, septi-, septo-**; **septic-, septico-**

septic-, septico-
denoting sepsis
combining form
From Greek **sēptikos** = putrefactive, from **sēpein** = to make rotten or putrid

septicaemia   blood poisoning caused by bacteria

! Do not confuse with ▸ **sept-, septi-, septem-**; **sept-, septi-, septo-**; **sept-, septo-**

septum
a partition or dividing structure in a cavity, tissue, etc
noun
From Latin **saeptum** = fence, wall, enclosure, from **saepire** = to enclose
Plural form **septa**

◆ Related words **septal** *or* **septate** *adj* ▸ partitioned

ser-, sero-
denoting serum
combining form
From Latin **serum** = whey, serum

seropositive	showing a serological reaction indicating the presence of a virus or disease, such as AIDS
seropurulent	containing a mixture of serum and pus, as in infected blisters
serotype	a group or category of bacteria or other micro-organisms that have a certain set of antigens in common or against which common antibodies are produced; the combination of antigens by which such a group is categorized

serous
relating to, resembling or consisting of serum
adjective
From medieval Latin **serosus**, from Latin **serum** = whey, serum

serous membrane	a serosa, a thin membrane, moist with serum, lining a cavity and enveloping the viscera within, such as the peritoneum or pericardium

seta
a bristle or a bristle-like structure
noun
From Latin **saeta** or **seta** = bristle
Plural form **setae**

setaceous
having bristles or bristle-like structures
adjective
From modern Latin **setaceus**, from Latin **saeta** or **seta** = bristle

! Do not confuse with ▸ **sebaceous**

sial-, sialo-
denoting saliva
combining form
From Greek **sialon** = saliva

sialagogue	anything that stimulates a flow of saliva
sialoid	resembling saliva
sialogram	an X-ray of the salivary tract
sialorrhoea	the excessive secretion of saliva

sider-, sidero-

denoting iron

combining form

From Greek **sidēros** = iron

sideropenia	iron deficiency
siderosis	a lung disease caused by breathing in iron or other metal particles

≈ Latin equivalent ▸**ferri-**

sinistr-, sinistro-

denoting on or to the left

combining form

From Latin **sinister**, genitive **sinistri** = on or to the left

sinistrocerebral	relating to or located on the left side of the brain
sinistrocular	having a dominant left eye

◐ Opposite ▸**dextr-, dextro-**

sino-

denoting a sinus

combining form

From Latin **sinus** = curve, fold, hollow, bay

sino-atrial node	a microscopic mass of specialized cardiac muscle in the right atrium of the heart, near the opening of the coronary sinus, that acts as the heart's pacemaker
sinopulmonary	relating to the paranasal sinuses and the lungs

sinus

a cavity or indentation in the body, such as the air-filled cavities in the bones of the skull, connecting with the nose (paranasal sinuses) or the dilations in the wall of the aorta above the cusps of the aortic valve (aortic sinuses); a narrow cavity through which pus is discharged; an abnormal communication between two hollow internal organs or between an internal organ and the exterior

noun

From Latin **sinus** = curve, fold, hollow, bay

Plural form **sinuses**

sinus-

denoting a sinus

combining form

From Latin **sinus** = curve, fold, hollow, bay

| **sinus**itis | inflammation of a sinus, especially one in the skull communicating with the nose |
| **sinus**oid | a small blood vessel in certain organs, such as the liver, heart, etc |

sito-
denoting food
combining form
From Greek **sitos** = grain, bread, food

| **sito**logy | the study of food, diet and nutrition |
| **sito**phobia | a pathological aversion to food |

skia-
denoting shadow
combining form
From Greek **skia** = shadow

| **skia**graph | an X-ray photograph |
| **skia**scopy | an examination of the eye by observing a shadow on the retina |

soma
the body, excluding the germ cells; the body as distinct from the mind
noun
From Greek **sōma**, genitive **sōmatos** = body
Plural form **somata** (or **somas**)

somat-, somato-
denoting the body; denoting a ▸ somatic cell; denoting the outer walls of the body
combining form
From Greek **sōma**, genitive **sōmatos** = body

somatogenic	originating in body cells
somatoplasm	the protoplasm of the somatic cells
somatosensory	relating to sensory stimuli perceived in the skin

somatic
relating to the body, excluding the germ cells; relating to the outer walls of the body, as distinct from the internal organs, the limbs and the head; relating to the body as distinct from the mind
adjective
From Greek **sōmatikos** = relating to the body, bodily, from **sōma**, genitive **sōmatos** = body

| **somatic** cell | one of the non-reproductive cells of the body, as distinct from the reproductive or germ cells |
| **somatic** mutation | a mutation occurring in somatic cells, and therefore not inheritable |

-somatic
denoting the body
combining form
From Greek **sōmatikos** = relating to the body, bodily, from **sōma**, genitive **sōmatos** = body

| psycho**somatic** | relating to the mind and body as a unit; concerned with or denoting physical diseases that have a psychological origin |

somato- see ▸ somat-, somato-

-some
denoting a body; denoting a chromosome
combining form
From Greek **sōma**, genitive **sōmatos** = body

auto**some**	a chromosome other than a sex chromosome
chromo**some**	any of the deeply staining rod-like structures seen in the nucleus at cell division
micro**some**	a minute granule or drop in cytoplasm

somn-, somni-, somno-
denoting sleep
combining form
From Latin **somnus** = sleep

somnambulism	sleepwalking
somnifacient	a drug that induces sleep
somniloquence	talking in one's sleep

≈ Greek equivalent ▸ **hypn-, hypno-**

-somnia
denoting sleep
combining form
From Latin **somnus** = sleep

| hyper**somnia** | a pathological tendency to sleep excessively |
| in**somnia** | sleeplessness |

sopor

unnaturally deep sleep

noun

From Latin **sopor** = deep sleep

soporific

inducing sleep

adjective

an agent that induces sleep

noun

From Latin **sopor** = deep sleep and **-ficus**, from **facere** = to do, to make

spasm

a sustained involuntary muscular contraction

noun

From Greek **spasmos** or **spasma** = spasm, convulsion, from **span** = to draw, to convulse

spasm-, spasmo-

denoting spasm

combining form

From Greek **spasmos** or **spasma** = spasm, convulsion, from **span** = to draw, to convulse

spasmolytic   a drug that alleviates spasms or convulsions

sphygm-, sphygmo-

denoting the pulse

combining form

From Greek **sphygmos** = pulsation, from **sphyzein** = to throb

sphygmograph   an instrument for recording the pulse, showing the rate and strength of the beats

sphygmoid   resembling a pulse

sphygmomano-meter   an instrument for measuring arterial blood pressure

sphygmus

the pulse

noun

From Greek **sphygmos** = pulsation, from **sphyzein** = to throb

◆ Related words **sphygmic** *adj* ▸relating to the pulse

spinal

relating to the backbone

adjective

From Latin **spinalis** = relating to the spine, spinal, from **spina** = thorn, backbone, spine

spinal canal	a passage running through the spinal column, containing the spinal cord
spinal column	the articulated series of vertebrae extending from the skull to the tip of the tail, forming the axis of the skeleton and enclosing the spinal cord
spinal cord	the main neural axis, consisting of a bundle of nerves running inside the spinal canal

spir-, spiro-[1]

denoting spiral, coil

combining form

From Latin **spira** = coil, from Greek **speira** = coil

spireme	in mitosis, the coiled thread formed by nuclear chromatin
spirillum	any rigid, spiral-shaped bacterium of the genus *Spirillum*, eg *S. minus* that causes rat-bite fever
spirochaete	a spirally coiled bacterium lacking a rigid cell wall, the cause of syphilis and other diseases

spir-, spiro-[2]

denoting breathing, respiration

combining form

From Latin **spirare** = to breathe

spirograph	an instrument for recording breathing movements
spirometer	an instrument for measuring lung capacity

-spiration

denoting breathing

combining form

From Latin **spirare** = to breathe

in**spiration**	breathing in
per**spiration**	the production and evaporation of sweat from the skin as a mechanism for excretion and cooling; the fluid thus produced

splanchn-, splanchno-

denoting the viscera or intestines

combining form

From Greek **splanchna** = innards, entrails, plural of **splanchnon**

splanchnocoele	a visceral cavity; the posterior part of the coelom
splanchnology	the study of the viscera

splanchnic

relating to the viscera or intestines
adjective
From Greek **splanchnikos** = relating to the bowels, from **splanchna** = innards, entrails, plural of **splanchnon**

splanchno- see ▸ splanchn-, splanchno-

splen-, spleno-

denoting the spleen
combining form
From Latin **splen**, genitive **splenis**, from Greek **splēn**, genitive **splēnos** = spleen

splenectomy	the surgical removal of the spleen
splenitis	inflammation of the spleen
splenomegaly	enlargement of the spleen

splenic

relating to the spleen
adjective
From Greek **splēnikos** = relating to the spleen, from **splēn**, genitive **splēnos** = spleen

spleno- see ▸ splen-, spleno-

spondyl-, spondylo-

denoting a vertebra or vertebrae
combining form
From Greek **sphondylos** or **spondylos** = vertebra

spondylitis	inflammation of the synovial joints of the backbone
spondylolisthesis	a partial dislocation of the vertebrae, usually the lower vertebrae, in which a vertebra slips forward over the one below
spondylolysis	the disintegration of one or more vertebrae
spondylosis	vertebral ankylosis
spondylosyndesis	surgical fusion of the joints between the vertebrae

squam-, squami-, squamo-

denoting scale; denoting the squamous portion of the temporal bone
combining form

From Latin **squama** = scale

squamiform	scalelike
squamocellular	relating to or consisting of flattened, scalelike cells
squamoparietal	relating to the squamous portion of the temporal bone and the parietal bone
squamosal	a paired membrane bone of the skull, the squamous portion of the temporal bone

squama

a scale; a scalelike structure; a thin plate of bone
noun
From Latin **squama** = scale
Plural form **squamae**

squami-, squamo- see ▸ squam-, squami-, squamo-

squamous

scaly; consisting of a layer of flattened scalelike cells
adjective
From Latin **squamosus** = scaly, from **squama** = scale

squamous cell carcinoma	a tumour of the flattened, scalelike cells in the skin

-stasis

denoting stoppage or stationariness
combining form
From Greek **stasis** = standing, stationariness, from **histanai** = to cause to stand, to stand

haemo**stasis**	stoppage of bleeding; stoppage or sluggishness of the circulation
homeo**stasis**	the tendency for the internal environment of the body to remain constant in spite of varying external conditions
meta**stasis**	the transfer of disease from its original site to another part of the body; a secondary tumour distant from the original site of disease

-static

denoting stopping or slowing something
combining form
From Greek **statikos** = causing to stand, bringing to a standstill, from **histanai** = to cause to stand, to stand

bacterio**static**	inhibiting the growth of bacteria
haemo**static**	stopping bleeding

status

a state or condition

noun

From Latin **status** = standing, position, state, condition, from **stare** = to stand

Plural form **status**

status asthmaticus	a severe, prolonged, potentially life-threatening asthma attack
status epilepticus	a condition in which someone has a series of epileptic seizures without recovering consciousness in the intervals between them

steat-, steato-

denoting fat or fatty tissue

combining form

From Greek **stear**, genitive **steatos** = hard fat, suet

steatocele	a fatty tumour in the scrotum
steatoma	a tumour of a sebaceous gland or sebaceous cyst
steatopygia	the accumulation of fat in the buttocks
steatorrhoea	the accumulation of abnormal levels of fat in the faeces

≈ Latin equivalent ▸ **adipo-**

sten-, steno-

denoting narrow, constricted, contracted

combining form

From Greek **stenos** = narrow

episio**sten**osis	a narrowing of the opening of the vulva
stenocephaly	abnormal narrowness of the head
stenosis	the constriction or narrowing of a tube or passage; constipation

sterc-, sterco-, stercor-, stercori-

denoting faeces

combining form

From Latin **stercus**, genitive **stercoris** = dung

stercolith	a hard mass of faeces
stercoraceous	relating to, consisting of, resembling or of the nature of faeces

≈ Greek equivalent ▸ **copr-, copro-**

stere-, stereo-

denoting solid, three-dimensional

combining form

From Greek **stereos** = firm, solid

stereoblind	having two-dimensional rather than normal three-dimensional vision
stereofluoroscope	a fluoroscope giving a three-dimensional view
stereognosis	the ability to perceive the three-dimensionality of a solid object by the sense of touch
stereoisomer	an isomer having the same chemical composition, molecular weight and structure, but differing spatial arrangement of atoms

stern-, sterno-
denoting the breastbone
combining form
From modern Latin **sternum**, from Greek **sternon** = chest, breast, breastbone

sternalgia	pain around the sternum, angina pectoris
sternebra	a segment of the breastbone
sternoclavicular	relating to the breastbone and collarbone
sternotomy	the surgical cutting of the breastbone

sternum
the breastbone
noun
From modern Latin **sternum**, from Greek **sternon** = chest, breast, breastbone
Plural form **sterna** (or **sternums**)
◆ Related words **sternal** *adj* ▸relating to the breastbone

steth-, stetho-
denoting the chest
combining form
From Greek **stēthos** = breast, chest

stethalgia	pain in the chest or pectoral muscles
stethoscope	an instrument with which to listen to the sounds produced by the heart, lungs, etc, with a hollow circular part that is applied to the body wall, from which sound is transmitted by tubes into earpieces
stethoparalysis	paralysis of the muscles of the chest

stom-, stomat-, stomato-
denoting the mouth; denoting an opening
combining form
From Greek **stoma**, genitive **stomatos** = mouth

anastomosis	a natural connection between two blood vessels; a surgical connection made between two hollow organs or parts
stomatitis	inflammation of the mucous membrane of the mouth
stomatodaeum	in embryology, the invagination that forms the anterior part of the digestive tract
stomatoplasty	plastic surgery of the mouth

≈ Latin equivalent ▸ **oro-**

stoma

the artificial opening of a tube that has been brought to the abdominal surface
noun
From Greek *stoma*, genitive *stomatos* = mouth
Plural form **stomata** (or **stomas**)

stomat-, stomato- see ▸ stom-, stomat-, stomato-

-stomy

denoting a surgical operation in which an opening is made in the specified organ or part
combining form
From Greek *-stomia*, from *stoma*, genitive *stomatos* = mouth

| colostomy | a surgical operation in which part of the colon is brought through an incision in the abdomen to form an artificial anus |
| gastrostomy | a surgical operation in which an opening is made in the stomach to introduce food into it |

! Do not confuse with ▸ **-tomy**

stratum

a layer of cells in living tissue
noun
From new Latin *stratum*, from Latin *stratum* = something spread out, from *stratus*, the past participle of *sternere* = to spread out
Plural form **strata**

stria

a fine streak, furrow or threadlike line, usually parallel to others
noun
From Latin *stria* = furrow, channel
Plural form **striae**

| **striae** gravidarum | stretch marks associated with pregnancy |

striated

marked with fine streaks, furrows or threadlike lines, usually parallel to one another

adjective

From Latin ***striatus*** = furrowed, channeled, from ***striare*** = to provide with furrows or channels

> **striated** muscle   a voluntary muscle or muscular tissue with fibres that are transversely striated

stroma

a supporting framework of connective tissue

noun

From Greek ***strōma***, genitive ***strōmatos*** = mattress, bed

Plural form **stromata**

◆ Related words **stromal** *adj* ▸relating to a supporting framework of connective tissue

sub-

denoting under, underneath, underlying, below; denoting part of, a subdivision of; denoting almost, partially, nearly, somewhat imperfectly, bordering on, deviating slightly from; denoting in smaller proportion

combining form

From Latin ***sub*** = under

> **sub**acute   not acute but progressing more rapidly than chronic
> **sub**cartilaginous   composed partly of cartilage; situated under a cartilage
> **sub**cellular   occurring within a cell; smaller than a cell
> **sub**clavian   situated or passing under the clavicle
> **sub**clinical disease   a disease that is not sufficiently developed to be detectable by usual clinical methods
> **sub**cutaneous   beneath or just under the skin
> **sub**luxation   partial dislocation or displacement, eg of a bone in a joint or a tooth in its socket

≈ Greek equivalent ▸ **hyp-, hypo-**

◑ Opposite ▸ **super-; supra-**

sudor

sweat

noun

From Latin ***sudor*** = sweat

◆ Related words **sudoral** *or* **sudorous** *adj* ▸relating to sweat; sweaty

sulcus

a groove or furrow, especially between two convolutions of the brain

noun

From Latin ***sulcus*** = furrow

Plural form **sulci**

◆ Related words **sulcal** *or* **sulcate** *adj* ▸relating to a groove or furrow, especially between two convolutions of the brain; grooved, furrowed

super-

denoting above or over; denoting beyond, exceeding, exceedingly, surpassing all others; denoting greater size, strength, extent, power, quantity, etc; denoting in addition, extra

combining form

From Latin ***super*** = above, over, on, in addition to

superbug	a strain of bacteria that is resistant to antibiotics
superciliary	relating to, on or near the eyebrow
supercoil	a complex coil formed by intertwining strands of protein or DNA
superinfection	an infection arising during and in addition to another infection and caused by a different micro-organism or a different variety of the same micro-organism
superovulation	the production of a larger number of ova than usual, eg under stimulus of injected hormones

≈ Greek equivalent ▸**hyper-**

◑ Opposite ▸**sub-**

superficial

relating to, on or near the surface

adjective

From Latin ***superficialis*** = relating to the surface, superficial, from ***superficies*** = surface, upper side, from ***super*** = above, over, on and ***facies*** = face, form, appearance

superior

upper or higher, especially in position

adjective

From Latin ***superior*** = upper, higher, comparative form of ***superus*** = situated above, upper, higher

superior vena cava	a vein that returns blood to the heart from the upper body

◑ Opposite ▸**inferior**

supine

lying face upwards; with the palm of the hand facing upwards
adjective
From Latin *supinus* = bent backwards, lying on the back
◖Opposite ▸**prone**

supra-

denoting above, over
combining form
From Latin *supra* = above, over, beyond

supraciliary	above the eyebrow
supracostal	above or on a rib
supraorbital	above the orbit of the eye
suprarenal	above the kidneys

≈ Greek equivalent ▸**hyper-**
◖Opposite ▸**sub-**

sy-, syl-, sym-, syn-, sys-

denoting together, with
combining form
From Greek *syn* = with

symbiosis	a mutually beneficial partnership between organisms of different kinds, especially where one lives on or within the other
symposium	an academic meeting at which research papers are presented (originally a drinking party)
syncytium	a multinucleate cell; a tissue without distinguishable cell membranes
syndactyly	a congenital condition in which the fingers or toes are fused together
syndrome	a concurrence of symptoms; a characteristic pattern or group of symptoms
syngeneic	genetically identical
systemic	relating to the bodily system or to a system of bodily organs; affecting the body as a whole

≈ Latin equivalent ▸**co-, com, con-**

sympath-, sympatho-

denoting a sympathetic nerve; denoting the sympathetic nervous system
combining form
From Greek *sympatheia* = sympathy, from *sympathēs* = sympathetic, from
syn = with and *pathos* = feeling, from *paschein* = to experience, to suffer

sympathectomy   the surgical removal of part of a sympathetic nerve
sympathomimetic a drug which mimics the action of the sympathetic
                     nervous system

---

sympathetic
relating to the sympathetic nervous system, the part of the autonomic
nervous system that controls the body's physiological responses to
dangerous or stressful situations
adjective
From Greek **sympatheia** = sympathy, from **sympathēs** = sympathetic, from
syn = with and **pathos** = feeling, from **paschein** = to experience, to suffer
   sympathetic   a nerve of the sympathetic nervous system
     nerve

---

sympatho- see ▸ sympath-, sympatho-

---

symptom
a subjective indication of a disease, ie something experienced by the patient,
not outwardly visible; any abnormal sensation, or emotional expression
or thought, accompanying a disease or disorder of the body or mind; any
objective evidence of disease or bodily disorder
noun
From Greek **symptōma**, genitive **symptōmatos** = chance, symptom, from
sympiptein = to happen to, from **syn** = with and **piptein** = to fall
◆ Related words **symptomatic** *adj* ▸relating to, constituting, showing or
involving a symptom or symptoms

---

syn- see ▸ sy-, syl-, sym, syn-, sys-

---

synapse
an interlacing or enveloping connection of one nerve cell with another
noun
From Greek **synapsis** = contact, junction, from **syn** = together and **haptein** = to
fasten, to join, to grasp, to touch
◆ Related words **synaptic** *adj* ▸relating to a synapse

---

syring-, syringo-
denoting a tube or tubular cavity, such as the Eustachian tube
combining form
From Greek **syrinx**, genitive **syringos** = shepherd's pipe, Pan pipes, passage, duct,
channel
   syringitis   inflammation of the Eustachian tube

syringomyelia   a chronic, progressive disease of the spinal cord in which tubular cavities develop within the cord, causing paralysis and loss of sensitivity to pain and temperature

---

sys- see ▸ **sy-, syl-, sym, syn-, sys-**

---

systole

rhythmical contraction, especially of the heart; the collapse of the nucleus in mitosis

noun

From Greek **systolē** = contraction, from **systellein** = to draw together, to contract, from **syn** = together and **stellein** = to prepare, to send

◆ Related words **systolic** *adj* ▸relating to rhythmical contraction, especially of the heart; relating to the collapse of the nucleus in mitosis

Tt

---

tachy-

denoting fast, rapid

combining form

From Greek **tachys** = fast

tachycardia	rapidity of heartbeat
tachyphasia	abnormally rapid or voluble speech
tachyphylaxis	a rapid build-up of tolerance to the effects of a drug
tachypnoea	abnormally rapid respiration

◑ Opposite ▸ **brady-**

-tactic

denoting movement of a cell or organism, eg a bacterium, in a definite direction in response to a stimulus

combining form

From Greek **taktikos** = relating to arrangement, disposition, order or position, from **tassein** = to marshal, to arrange

chemo**tactic**	relating to the movement of a cell or organism in a definite direction in response to chemical stimulus
hydro**tactic**	relating to the movement of a cell or organism in a definite direction in response to the stimulus of water

---

tactile

perceptible by touch; relating to the sense of touch; concerned with perception by touch

adjective
From Latin ***tactilis*** = touchable, tangible, from ***tangere*** = to touch

tal-, tali-, talo-
denoting the ankle bone
combining form
From Latin ***talus*** = ankle, ankle bone, heel

talalgia	pain in the ankle
talipes	club foot
talofibular	relating to the ankle bone and the fibula

talus
the ankle bone or astragalus
noun
From Latin ***talus*** = ankle, ankle bone, heel
Plural form **tali**

tarsus
the bones forming the part of the foot to which the leg is articulated; a plate of connective tissue at the edge of the eyelid
noun
From modern Latin ***tarsus***, from Greek ***tarsos*** = flat of the foot, ankle, edge of the eyelid and its lashes
Plural form **tarsi**

-tarsus
denoting the tarsus of the foot
combining form
From modern Latin ***tarsus***, from Greek ***tarsos*** = flat of the foot, ankle, edge of the eyelid and its lashes
Plural form **-tarsi**

meta**tarsus**	the part of the foot between the tarsus and the toes

taxis
the return to position of displaced parts by means of manipulation only; the movement of a cell or organism, eg a bacterium, in a definite direction in response to a stimulus
noun
From Greek ***taxis*** = arrangement, disposition, order, position, from ***tassein*** = to marshal, to arrange
Plural form **taxes**

-taxis

denoting movement in response to stimulus

combining form

From Greek ***taxis*** = arrangement, disposition, order, position, from ***tassein*** = to marshal, to arrange

Plural form **-taxes**

chemo**taxis**	the movement of a cell or organism in a definite direction in response to chemical stimulus
hydro**taxis**	the movement of a cell or organism in a definite direction in response to the stimulus of water

tel-, tele-

denoting far, distant, over a distance; denoting television; denoting telecommunications

combining form

From Greek ***tēle*** = far

telemedicine	the use of telecommunications technology to transmit medical advice, diagnoses, etc

! Do not confuse with ▸ **tel-, telo-**

tel-, telo-

denoting end, completion

combining form

From Greek ***telos*** = end

telangiectasis	a dilatation of the small arteries or capillaries
telomere	the structure which terminates the arm of a chromosome, protecting the chromosome against gene loss and decay
telophase	in mitosis, the stage of reconstruction of nuclei after separation of daughter chromosomes

! Do not confuse with ▸ **tel-, tele-**

tempo-, temporo-

denoting time; denoting temple; denoting temporal lobe

combining form

From Latin ***tempus***, genitive ***temporis*** = time, temple

tempolabile	tending to change with time
temporo-mandibular	relating to the temporal bone and the mandible
temporopontile	relating to the temporal lobe and the pons of the brain

temporal

relating to time; relating to or close to the temples on either side of the head

adjective

From Latin ***temporalis*** = relating to time, temporal; relating to the temples, temporal, from ***tempus***, genitive ***temporis*** = time, temple

temporal bone	either of a pair of bones that form part of the sides and base of the skull and contain the middle and inner ears
temporal summation	the summation of successive stimuli over a short period of time; for example, repeated small stimulations of a neuron causing it to fire when one such stimulation would be inadequate

temporo- see ▶ **tempor-, temporo-**

ten-, teno-

denoting a tendon

combining form

From Greek ***tenōn***, genitive ***tenontos*** = sinew, tendon

tenalgia	pain in a tendon
tenorrhaphy	the surgical repair of a split or torn tendon by an operation involving suturing
tenosynovitis	painful inflammation and swelling of a tendon, associated with repetitive movements

-tene

denoting a ribbon, band or thread

combining form

From Greek ***taenia*** = band

pachy**tene**	a stage of meiosis during which the chromosomes become thick and the individual chromatids can be distinguished

terat-, terato-

denoting monster, congenital malformation

combining form

From Greek ***teras***, genitive ***teratos*** = monster, monstrosity

teratogen	an agent that raises the incidence of congenital malformation
teratology	the study of biological malformations or abnormal growths
teratoma	a tumour consisting of tissue not normally found at that site, occurring especially in the testis or ovary

testis
> a testicle
> *noun*
> From Latin ***testis*** = witness, testicle ('witness of virility')
> Plural form **testes**

tetr-, tetra-
> denoting four
> *combining form*
> From Greek ***tetra-*** = four-, from ***tettares*** or ***tessares*** = four
>
> | **tetra**dactyly | a congenital condition in which someone has only four fingers or toes |
> | **tetra**plegia | paralysis of all four limbs |
> | **tetra**ploid | having four sets of chromosomes |
>
> ≈ Latin equivalent ▸ **quadr-, quadri-**

thalam-, thalamo-
> denoting the thalamus
> *combining form*
> From Greek ***thalamos*** = inner room, bedroom
>
> | **thalam-** encephalon | the part of the diencephalon that includes the pineal gland and thalamus |
> | **thalamo**tomy | a surgical incision into the thalamus |

thalamus
> either of the two parts of the midbrain where the optic nerve emerges
> *noun*
> From Greek ***thalamos*** = inner room, bedroom
> Plural form **thalami**

-thalamus
> denoting the thalamus
> *combining form*
> From Greek ***thalamos*** = inner room, bedroom
> Plural form **-thalami**
>
> | hypo**thalamus** | a part of the brain that lies under the thalamus |

theca
> a sheath, case or sac
> *noun*
> From Latin ***theca***, from Greek ***thēkē*** = case, sheath
> Plural form **thecae**

-thecal

denoting a case, sheath, sac

combining form

From Latin ***theca***, from Greek ***thēkē*** = case, sheath

intra**thecal**	within or introduced into the sheath of the spinal cord or brain

-thelium

denoting cell tissue

combining form

From Greek ***thēlē*** = nipple

endo**thelium**	the layer of cell tissue on the internal surfaces of blood vessels, lymphatics, etc
epi**thelium**	cell tissue that covers the outer surface of the body or mucous membranes connected with it, or lines the closed cavities of the body
meso**thelium**	cell tissue that forms the lining of the pleural, pericardial and peritoneal cavities and that lines the body cavity of an embryo

therm-, thermo-

denoting heat

combining form

From Greek ***thermos*** = hot or ***thermē*** = heat

thermogenesis	the production of heat in the body by physiological processes
thermography	an image of heat emission from the patient's body used in medical diagnosis, eg for detecting tumours
thermometer	an instrument for measuring temperature

-thermia

denoting temperature

combining form

From Greek ***thermē*** = heat

hyper**thermia**	abnormally high body temperature
hypo**thermia**	abnormally low body temperature, caused by exposure to cold or induced for the purpose of heart and other surgery

-thermic

denoting temperature

combining form

thermo-

From Greek **thermē** = heat

poikilo**thermic**   having a variable blood-temperature, cold-blooded

thermo- see ▸ therm-, thermo-

thora-, thorac-, thoraco-
denoting the ▸ **thorax**

combining form

From Greek **thōrax**, genitive **thōrakos** = breastplate, trunk, chest

thoracocentesis   the puncturing of the pleural cavity through the chest wall with a hollow needle to withdraw fluid, blood or air

thoracostomy   the construction of an artificial opening in the chest, usually to draw off fluid or release a build-up of air

thoracotomy   a surgical incision into the wall of the chest, for drawing pus from the pleural cavity or lung

thoracic
relating to or located in or near the thorax

noun

From Greek **thōrakikos** = relating to the chest, suffering in the chest, from **thōrax**, genitive **thōrakos** = breastplate, trunk, chest

thoracic duct   the main trunk of the vessels conveying lymph in the body

thoraco- see ▸ thora-, thorac-, thoraco-

thorax
the part of the body between the head and abdomen, the chest

noun

From Greek **thōrax**, genitive **thōrakos** = breastplate, trunk, chest

Plural form **thoraces** (or **thoraxes**)

-thrix
denoting hair or something resembling hair

combining form

From Greek **thrix**, genitive **trichos** = hair

endo**thrix**   a parasitic fungus affecting the inner part of the shaft of the hair

monile**thrix**   a condition in which the hair has a large number of constrictions that look like tiny beads, does not grow very long and breaks easily

thromb-, thrombo-
denoting a clot or clotting

combining form

From Greek ***thrombos*** = lump, clot

thrombocyte	a platelet
thrombocytopenia	an abnormal decrease in the number of platelets in the blood, causing haemorrhage
thrombolysis	the dissolving of clots in the blood
thrombosis	the inappropriate clotting of blood within a vessel

thrombus
a clot of blood in a living vessel, obstructing circulation

noun

From Greek ***thrombos*** = lump, clot

Plural form **thrombi**

thym-, thymo-
denoting the thymus

combining form

From Greek ***thymos*** = wart, thymus gland

thymectomy	the surgical removal of the thymus
thymocyte	an immature lymphocyte found in the thymus, the precursor of the T-lymphocyte

thymus
a ductless gland near the root of the neck, producing white blood cells at early ages but vestigial in adults

noun

From Greek ***thymos*** = wart, thymus gland

Plural form **thymi** (or **thymuses**)

◆ Related words **thymic** *adj* ▸relating to the thymus

thyr-, thyro-
denoting the thyroid gland

combining form

From Greek ***thyreoeidēs*** = shield-shaped, thyroid, from ***thyreos*** = oblong shield shaped like a door, from ***thyra*** = door and ***-oeidēs*** = resembling, having the form of, from ***eidos*** = form, shape

thyrotoxicosis	a disease condition resulting from excessive activity of the thyroid gland
thyrotrop(h)in	a hormone, produced in the anterior lobe of the pituitary gland, which stimulates the thyroid gland

thyroid

relating to the thyroid gland or the thyroid cartilage
adjective
the thyroid gland; the thyroid cartilage
noun
From Greek **thyreoeidēs** = shield-shaped, thyroid, from **thyreos** = oblong shield shaped like a door, from **thyra** = door and **-oeidēs** = resembling, having the form of, from **eidos** = form, shape

thyroid cartilage	the principal cartilage of the larynx, forming the Adam's apple
thyroid gland	a ductless gland in the neck that secretes thyroxin

tibia

the shinbone, the thicker of the two bones of the leg below the knee
noun
From Latin **tibia** = shinbone, shin, pipe, flute
Plural form **tibiae** (or **tibias**)
◆ Related words **tibial** *adj* ▸relating to the shinbone

tibi-, tibio-

denoting the tibia
combining form
From Latin **tibia** = shinbone, shin, pipe, flute

tibialgia	pain in the tibia
tibiofibular	relating to the tibia and the fibula

toc-, toco-, tok-, toko-

denoting childbirth
combining form
From Greek **tokos** = childbirth, offspring, from **tiktein** = to father, to give birth to

cardio**toco**graphy	the recording of the fetal heart rate by means of an electronic instrument
dys**toc**ia	abnormal or difficult labour or childbirth
tocology	obstetrics

-tomy

denoting surgical cutting or incision
combining form
From Greek **tomē** = cutting, cut, from **temnein** = to cut

amnio**tomy**	the cutting of the amnion to induce labour
ana**tomy**	the science of the structure of the human body, learned by cutting it up

| episio**tomy** | an incision made in the perineum to facilitate the delivery of a baby |
| thoraco**tomy** | a surgical incision into the wall of the chest, for drawing pus from the pleural cavity or lung |

! Do not confuse with ▸ **-stomy**

---

ton-, tono-

denoting tension, tone, pressure

combining form

From Greek ***tonos*** = tension, tone from ***teinein*** = to stretch

| dys**ton**ia | a disorder of muscle tone, causing muscle spasm |
| **tono**meter | an instrument for measuring fluid pressure (eg within the eyeball) or blood pressure |

---

tonic

producing tension of the muscles; giving tone and vigour to the system

adjective

a medicine that invigorates and strengthens

noun

From Greek ***tonikos*** = relating to stretching, capable of extension, contractile, from ***tonos*** = tension, tone from ***teinein*** = to stretch

| **tonic** spasm | a prolonged uniform muscular spasm |

◆ Related words **tonicity** *n* the healthy elasticity of muscular fibres when at rest

---

-tonic

denoting tension, pressure, concentration

combining form

From Greek ***tonikos*** = relating to stretching, capable of extension, contractile, from ***tonos*** = tension, tone from ***teinein*** = to stretch

| iso**tonic** | having the same muscle tension; having the same osmotic pressure; containing salts and minerals of the same concentration as in the body |

---

tono- see ▸ **ton-, tono-**

---

top-, topo-

denoting place

combining form

From Greek ***topos*** = place

| **top**agnosis | the inability to identify a part of the body that has been touched as a result of disease of or damage to the brain |

topognosis	the ability to identify a part of the body that has been touched
topography	the detailed study or description of external features of the body with reference to those underneath
topology	the anatomy of a particular part or area of the body

-topia

denoting place

combining form

From Greek **topos** = place

| ec**topia** | the abnormal displacement of an organ or part |

-topic

denoting place

combining form

From Greek **topikos** = relating to a place, local, topical, from **topos** = place

| ec**topic** | in an abnormal position |
| hetero**topic** | displaced |

topo- see ▸ top-, topo-

-topy

denoting place

combining form

From Greek **topos** = place

| hetero**topy** | the displacement of an organ of the body or the presence of normal tissue at an abnormal site |

trachea

a passage strengthened by cartilaginous rings that carries air from the larynx to the bronchi, the windpipe

noun

From medieval Latin **trachea**, from Greek **tracheia (artēriā)** = rough (windpipe), from **trachys, tracheia, trachy** = rough

Plural form **tracheae** (or **tracheas**)

◆ Related words **tracheal** *adj* ▸relating to the windpipe

tra-, tran-, trans-

across, beyond, through

combining form

From Latin **trans** = across, over, beyond, through

| **trans**dermal | absorbed or injected through the skin |

translocation	the transfer of a portion of a chromosome to another part of the same chromosome or to a different chromosome, with or without loss of genetic material
transplant	the surgical removal of a part or organ from its normal position and the grafting of it into another position in the same individual or into another individual; the organ, tissue, etc transplanted
transsexual	a person anatomically of one sex but having a strong desire to adopt the physical characteristics and role of a member of the opposite sex; a person who has had medical and surgical treatment to alter the external sexual features so that they resemble those of the opposite sex
transudate	a fluid that passes through a membrane or the walls of a blood vessel
transverse colon	the part of the colon lying across the abdominal cavity

tract

a region of the body occupied by a particular system

noun

From Latin ***tractus*** = drawing, dragging, pulling, tract, region, from ***trahere*** = to draw, to drag, to pull

tran-, trans- see ▸ tra-, tran-, trans-

trauma

an injury (*med*); an emotional shock that may be the origin of a neurosis (*psych*); the state or condition caused by a physical or emotional shock

noun

From Greek ***trauma***, genitive ***traumatos*** = wound

Plural form **traumata** (or **traumas**)

◆ Related words **traumatic** *adj* ▸relating to, resulting from or causing injury (*med*); relating to, resulting from or causing a lasting emotional shock (*psych*)

tri-

denoting three, threefold

combining form

From Latin ***tres***, ***tria*** and Greek ***treis***, ***tria*** = three

trigeminal nerve	a facial nerve with three branches, supplying the eye, nose, skin, scalp and muscles of mastication
trimester	a three-month period of a pregnancy
trisomy	a condition in which a chromosome occurs three times in a cell instead of twice

trich-, tricho-
denoting hair
combining form
From Greek ***thrix***, genitive ***trichos*** = hair

trichiasis	the turning in of hairs around an orifice, especially of eyelashes so that they rub against the eye
trichoid	hairlike
trichotillomania	a neurosis in which the patient pulls out tufts of his or her own hair

trop-, tropo-
denoting turning
combining form
From Greek ***tropos*** = turn, from ***trepein*** = to turn

tropomyosin	a filamentous protein that controls the interaction of actin and myosin in muscle fibres, and hence muscle contraction

! Do not confuse with ▸ **troph-, tropho-**

troph-, tropho-
denoting nutrition
combining form
From Greek ***trophē*** = nourishment, food, from ***trephein*** = to feed, to nourish, to rear

trophoblast	the outer layer of a mammalian blastocyst, which supplies nutrients to the developing embryo
trophology	the study of nutrition

! Do not confuse with ▸ **trop-, tropo-**

-trophic
denoting nutrition, growth; denoting stimulation
combining form
From Greek ***trophikos*** = nursing, alimentary, from ***trophē*** = nourishment, food, from ***trephein*** = to feed, to nourish, to rear

eu**trophic**	relating to healthy nutrition
gonado**trophic**	stimulating the gonads
neuro**trophic**	relating to the nutrition of the nervous system, or to nutritional changes influenced by the nervous system

! Do not confuse with ▸ **-tropic**

tropho- see ▸ **troph-, tropho-**

-trophy

denoting nutrition, growth; denoting stimulation
combining form
From Greek **-trophia**, from **trophē** = nourishment, food, from **trephein** = to feed, to nourish, to rear

a**trophy**	wasting away or diminution of size and functional activity of a body part or tissue
muscular dys**trophy**	any of several disorders in which there is progressive wasting of muscle tissue
hyper**trophy**	overnourishment of an organ etc, causing abnormal enlargement

-tropic

denoting turning; denoting tendency towards or affinity for the specified thing
combining form
From Greek **tropikos**, from **tropos** = turn, from **trepein** = to turn

neuro**tropic**	having a special affinity for or growing in nerve cells
psycho**tropic** drug	a drug that affects the brain and influences behaviour, heightens sensitivity, etc

! Do not confuse with ▸ **-trophic**

tropo- see ▸ trop-, tropo-

tub-, tubo-

denoting tube, especially a Fallopian tube or the Eustachian tube
combining form
From Latin **tubus** = pipe, tube

tubectomy	the surgical removal of a Fallopian tube
tubo-abdominal	relating to or developing in a Fallopian tube and the abdominal cavity
tuboplasty	the surgical repair of a Fallopian tube
tubotympanic	relating to the Eustachian tube and the tympanic cavity

≈ Greek equivalent ▸ **salping-, salpingo-**

tunica

a membrane or layer that covers or lines an organ or other structure
noun
From Latin **tunica** = tunic
Plural form **tunicae**

turgor

the state of being swollen, usually because of a build-up of fluid

noun

From Latin **turgor** = swelling, from **turgere** = to swell, to be swollen

◆ Related words **turgid** *adj* ▹swollen, usually because of a build-up of fluid

tussis

a cough or coughing

noun

From Latin **tussis** = cough

Plural form **tusses**

◆ Related words **tussive** *adj* ▹relating to or caused by a cough or coughing

tympan-, tympano-

denoting the middle ear; denoting the eardrum; denoting swollen shape

combining form

From Greek **tympanon** or **typanon** = kettledrum, from **typtein** = to beat, to strike

tympanectomy	the surgical removal of the eardrum
tympanites	flatulent distension of the belly
tympanitis	inflammation of the membrane of the ear
tympano-eustachian	relating to the middle ear and the Eustachian tube

tympanic

relating to the middle ear; relating to the eardrum; relating to or affected with tympanites, a flatulant distension of the belly

adjective

a bone of the ear, supporting the drum membrane

noun

From Greek **tympanon** or **typanon** = kettledrum, from **typtein** = to beat, to strike

tympanic bone	a bone of the ear, supporting the drum membrane
tympanic membrane	the membrane separating the middle ear from the outer ear

tympano- see ▸ tympan-, tympano-

tympanum

the middle ear; the membrane separating the middle ear from the outer ear, the eardrum or tympanic membrane

noun

From Greek **tympanon** or **typanon** = kettledrum, from **typtein** = to beat, to strike

Plural form **tympana** (or **tympanums**)

Uu

ul-, ule-, ulo-
   denoting a scar or scar tissue
   combining form
   From Greek ***oulē*** = scar

     ulegyria   a condition in which scarring from lesions in the fetus or infant causes the gyri of the brain to become narrow and distorted

     ulosis   the formation of a scar

   ! Do not confuse with ▸**ul-, ulo-**

---

ul-, ulo-
   denoting the gums
   combining form
   From Greek ***oulon*** = gum

     ulitis   inflammation of the gums, gingivitis

   ! Do not confuse with ▸**ul-, ule-, ulo-**

---

ulna
   the inner and larger of the two bones of the forearm
   noun
   From Latin ***ulna*** = elbow, arm
   Plural form **ulnae** (or **ulnas**)
   ◆ Related words **ulnar** *adj* ▸relating to the ulna

---

ulo- see ▸**ul-, ulo-**; **ul-, ule-, ulo-**

---

ultra-
   denoting beyond; denoting to an extreme degree
   combining form
   From Latin ***ultra*** = beyond

     ultracentrifuge   a high-speed centrifuge
     ultrafiltration   the separation of particles by filtration, under suction or pressure
     ultrasound   sound waves or vibrations too rapid to be audible, used in medical diagnosis

---

umbilical
   relating to the umbilicus or the umbilical cord
   adjective

the umbilical cord

noun

From Latin ***umbilicus*** = navel

umbilical cord   a long flexible tube connecting the fetus to the placenta

≈ Greek equivalent ▸ **omphalic**

---

umbilicus

the navel

noun

From Latin ***umbilicus*** = navel

Plural form **umbilici** (or **umbilicuses**)

---

uni-

denoting one

combining form

From Latin ***unus*** = one

unicellular	relating to or having only one cell
unilateral	relating to, located on or affecting only one side of the body or of an organ
uniparous	having given birth to only one child

≈ Greek equivalent ▸ **mon-, mono-**

---

ur-, uro-

denoting urine

combining form

From Greek ***ouron*** = urine

uraemia	the retention in the blood of waste materials normally excreted in urine, particulary urea
urogenital	relating to the urinary and sexual functions or organs
urology	the study of the diseases and abnormalities of the urinary tract and their treatment
uropoiesis	the formation of urine

≈ Latin equivalent ▸ **urin-, urini-, urino-**

---

uran-, urano-

denoting the roof of the mouth, palate

combining form

From Greek ***ouranos*** = heaven, sky, roof of the mouth, palate

uraniscus	the roof of the mouth
uranoplasty	plastic surgery of the palate

! Do not confuse with ▸**urin-, urini-, urino-**
≈ Latin equivalent ▸**palato-**

-uresis

denoting urination
combining form
From Greek ***ourēsis*** = urination, from ***ourein*** = to urinate, from ***ouron*** = urine

di**uresis**	increased or excessive excretion of urine
en**uresis**	involuntary urination, especially while asleep
natri**uresis**	the excretion of sodium in the urine

-uretic

denoting urination
combining form
From Greek ***ourētikos*** = urinating a lot or frequently, promoting or resembling urine, from ***ourein*** = to urinate, from ***ouron*** = urine

di**uretic**	increasing the flow of urine (*adj*); a medicine or other substance that increases the flow of urine (*n*)
natri**uretic**	relating to, characterized by or promoting the excretion of sodium in the urine

---

-uria

denoting urination of a specified type; denoting the presence in the urine of the specified substance
combining form
From Greek **-*ouria***, from ***ouron*** = urine

dys**uria**	difficulty or pain in urinating
haemat**uria**	the presence of blood in the urine
melan**uria**	the presence of melanin pigments in the urine
poly**uria**	excessive secretion of urine

---

urin-, urini-, urino-

denoting urine
combining form
From Latin ***urina*** = urine

urinalysis	the analysis of urine, eg to detect disease
uriniparous	producing urine
urinogenital	relating jointly to urinary and genital functions or organs
urinometer	an instrument for measuring the specific gravity of urine

! Do not confuse with ▸**uran-, urano-**
≈ Greek equivalent ▸**ur-, uro-**

urinary

relating to or resembling urine, or the organs that produce urine

adjective

From Latin ***urina*** = urine

---

urini-, urino- see ▸ urin-, urini-, urino-

---

uro- see ▸ ur-, uro-

---

uter-, utero-

denoting the uterus, womb

combining form

From Latin ***uterus*** = womb

uteritis	inflammation of the womb
uterectomy	the surgical removal of the uterus, hysterectomy
uterogestation	gestation in the womb
uterotomy	a surgical incision of the uterus

---

uterine

relating to, in or for the uterus; having the same mother but a different father

adjective

From Latin ***uterinus*** = having the same mother, uterine, from ***uterus*** = womb

---

-uterine

denoting the uterus, womb

combining form

From Latin ***uterinus*** = having the same mother, uterine, from ***uterus*** = womb

extra**uterine**	outside the uterus
intra**uterine**	within the uterus

---

utero- see ▸ uter-, utero-

---

uterus

the womb

noun

From Latin ***uterus*** = womb

Plural form **uteri** (or **uteruses**)

Vv

vag-, vago-
denoting the ▸ **vagus** or **vagus nerve**

combining form

From Latin ***vagus*** = wandering

vagectomy	the surgical removal of all or part of the vagus
vagotomy	a surgical incision into the vagus, especially to reduce gastric secretion

vagus or vagus nerve
the tenth cranial nerve, concerned with regulating heartbeat, rhythm of breathing, etc

noun

From Latin ***vagus*** = wandering

Plural form **vagi**

valgus
displaced from normal alignment so as to deviate away from the midline of the body

adjective

From Latin ***valgus*** = bow-legged

varus
displaced from normal alignment so as to deviate towards the midline of the body

adjective

From Latin ***varus*** = bent inwards, knock-kneed

vas
a vessel, tube or duct carrying liquid

noun

From Latin ***vas***, genitive ***vasis*** = vessel

Plural form **vasa**

vas deferens	the spermatic duct, carrying spermatozoa from the testis to the urethra

vas-, vaso-
denoting blood vessels; denoting the vas deferens

combining form

From Latin ***vas***, genitive ***vasis*** = vessel

vasectomy	the surgical removal of part or all of the vas deferens, especially in order to produce sterility
vasoactive	promoting the narrowing or expansion of blood vessels
vasodilation	the expansion of a blood vessel

vascul-, vasculo-

denoting blood vessels

combining form

From Latin ***vasculum*** = small vessel

vasculitis	inflammation of a blood vessel
vasculolymphatic	relating to blood vessels and lymphatic vessels
vasculopathy	a disease of the blood vessels

vascular

relating to, composed of or provided with blood vessels

adjective

From modern Latin ***vascularis***, from Latin ***vasculum*** = small vessel

| **vascular** disease | any of various diseased conditions of the blood vessels |

-vascular

denoting blood vessels

combining form

From modern Latin ***vascularis***, from Latin ***vasculum*** = small vessel

cardio**vascular**	relating to the heart and blood vessels
cerebro**vascular**	relating to the brain and its blood vessels
extra**vascular**	located or occurring outside the vascular system or a blood vessel
neuro**vascular**	relating to or affecting both nerves and blood vessels

vasculo- see ▶ vascul-, vasculo-

vaso- see ▶ vas-, vaso-

vena

a vein

noun

From Latin ***vena*** = blood vessel, vein, artery

Plural form **venae**

| **vena** cava | either of the two major veins taking venous blood to the heart |

vene-, veni-, veno-

denoting a vein

combining form

From Latin **vena** = blood vessel, vein, artery

venepuncture — the puncturing of a vein with a hypodermic needle, to draw off a sample of blood or inject a drug

venography — the radiography of a vein after injection of a contrast medium

≈ Greek equivalent ▸ **phleb-, phlebo-**

venous

relating to or contained in veins; full of veins; deoxygenated and dark red in colour

adjective

From Latin **venosus** = full of veins, veiny, from **vena** = blood vessel, vein, artery

venous blood — blood in the veins that is deoxygenated and dark red in colour

-venous

denoting a vein

combining form

From Latin **venosus** = full of veins, veiny, from **vena** = blood vessel, vein, artery

intra**venous** — within or introduced into a vein or veins

ventral

relating to the abdomen; relating to the front of the body or an organ

adjective

From Latin **ventralis** = relating to the belly, from **venter**, genitive **ventris** = belly

◑ Opposite ▸ **dorsal**

ventricle

either of the two lower contractile chambers of the heart, the right ventricle receiving venous blood from the right atrium and pumping it into the pulmonary loop for oxygenation, the left receiving oxygenated blood from the left atrium and pumping it into the arterial system for circulation round the body; any of various other cavities in the body, eg one of the four main cavities of the brain

noun

From Latin **ventriculus** = belly, ventricle, from **venter**, genitive **ventris** = belly

ventricular

relating to or of the nature of a ventricle; abdominal

adjective

From Latin **ventriculus** = belly, ventricle, from **venter**, genitive **ventris** = belly

ventricular   uncoordinated rapid electric activity of a heart ventricle
    fibrillation

-ventricular

relating to the abdomen; relating to the front of the body or an organ

combining form

From Latin **ventriculus** = belly, ventricle, from **venter**, genitive **ventris** = belly

atrio**ventricular**   relating to the atria and ventricles of the heart

---

verruca

a wart, especially one on the sole of the foot

noun

From Latin **verruca** = wart

Plural form **verrucae** (or **verrucas**)

---

vertebra

any of the segments that compose the backbone

noun

From Latin **vertebra** = joint, vertebra, from **vertere** = to turn

Plural form **vertebrae**

---

vertebral

relating to vertebrae

adjective

From Latin **vertebra** = joint, vertebra, from **vertere** = to turn

vertebral column   the spinal column

---

vertigo

dizziness, giddiness; a whirling sensation experienced when the sense of
balance is disturbed

noun

From Latin **vertigo**, genitive **vertiginis** = turning round, whirling round, dizziness,
giddiness, from **vertere** = to turn

Plural form **vertigines** (or **vertigoes** or **vertigos**)

---

vesic-, vesico-

denoting the urinary bladder

combining form

From Latin **vesica** = bladder, blister

vesicorenal   relating to the urinary bladder and the kidneys

vesicovaginal   relating to the urinary bladder and the vagina

≈ Greek equivalent ▸ **cyst-, cysto-**

vesica

a bladder or sac, especially the urinary bladder

noun

From Latin **vesica** = bladder, blister

Plural form **vesicae**

◆ Related words **vesical** *adj* ▸relating to a bladder or sac, especially the urinary bladder

vesicle

a small globule, bladder, sac, blister, cavity, or swelling; a primary cavity of the brain

noun

From Latin **vesicula** = little blister, vesicle, from **vesica** = bladder, blister

◆ Related words **vesicular** *adj* ▸relating to a vesicle

vesico- see ▸ vesic-, vesico-

vestigial

relating to or existing as a reduced and functionless structure, organ, etc, representing what was once useful and developed

adjective

From Latin **vestigium** = footprint, trace, vestige

villus

a hairlike process, especially one of the frond-like extensions of the lining of the small intestine

noun

From Latin **villus** = shaggy hair, tuft of hair

Plural form **villi**

viscera

the organs situated within the chest and the abdomen, heart, lungs, liver, etc, especially the abdominal organs

noun

From Latin **viscera** = internal organs, viscera, plural of **viscus**, genitive **visceris**

Singular form **viscus**

◆ Related words **visceral** *adj* ▸relating to the organs situated within the chest and the abdomen, heart, lungs, liver, etc, especially the abdominal organs

vision

the faculty of sight

noun

From Latin **visio**, genitive **visionis** seeing, sight, vision, from **videre** = to see

visual

relating to sight or seeing

adjective

From Latin ***visualis*** = attained by sight, from ***visus*** seeing, sight, vision, from ***videre*** = to see

visual acuity	the spatial resolving power of the eye
visual field	the area visible to an observer at any one time

vita

life

noun

From Latin ***vita*** = life

Plural form **vitae** (or **vitas**)

vital

relating to or characteristic of life or of living things; supporting or necessary to life

adjective

From Latin ***vitalis*** = relating to life, vital, from ***vita*** = life

vital capacity	the volume of air that can be expelled from the lungs after taking the deepest possible breath
vital functions	the bodily functions that are essential to life, such as the circulation of the blood
vital signs	(the level or rate of) breathing, heartbeat, etc
vital stain	a stain that can be used on living cells without killing them

vitreous

glassy; relating to, consisting of or resembling glass

adjective

From Latin ***vitreus*** = made of glass, resembling glass, glassy, from ***vitrum*** = glass

vitreous humour	the jellylike substance filling the posterior chamber of the eye, between the lens and the retina

-volaemia

denoting blood volume

combining form

From volume and Greek ***-aimia***, from ***haima*** = blood

hyper**volaemia**	an abnormally high volume of blood circulating in the body
hypo**volaemia**	an abnormally low volume of blood circulating in the body

vulnerary

relating to wounds; useful in healing wounds

adjective

a drug or medicine used for healing wounds

noun

From Latin ***vulneraruis*** = relating to wounds, from ***vulnus***, genitive ***vulneris*** = wound

vulv-, vulvo-

denoting the vulva

combining form

From Latin ***volva*** or ***vulva*** = wrapper, covering, womb

vulvitis	inflammation of the vulva
vulvo-uterine	relating to the vulva and the uterus

vulva

the external genitals of the human female, especially the orifice of the vagina

noun

From Latin ***volva*** or ***vulva*** = wrapper, covering, womb

Plural form **vulvae** (or **vulvas**)

◆▸ Related words **vulval**, **vulvar** *or* **vulvate** *adj* ▸relating to the vulva

vulvo- see ▸ **vulv-, vulvo-**

Xx

xanth-, xantho-

denoting yellow

combining form

From Greek ***xanthos*** = yellow

xanthochromia	any yellowish discoloration, especially of the cerebrospinal fluid
xanthoma	a yellow tumour composed of fibrous tissue and of cells containing cholesterol ester, occurring on the skin (eg in diabetes) or on the sheaths of tendons, or in any tissue of the body
xanthopsia	a condition in which objects appear yellow to the observer, as in jaundice

xen-, xeno-
denoting foreign, different
combining form
From Greek ***xenos*** = foreign, strange

xenobiotic	denoting or relating to a substance foreign to or not rightly found in a body, biological system, etc
xenogenic	due to an outside cause
xenograft	a graft from a member of a different species
xenotransplant-ation	the transplanting of an organ from an individual of one species into an individual of another species

xer-, xero-
denoting dry
combining form
From Greek ***xēros*** = dry

xeroderma	a disease characterized by abnormal dryness of the skin and by abnormal excessive growth of its horny layer
xerophthalmia	a dry lustreless condition of the conjunctiva as a result of a deficiency of vitamin A in the diet
xerosis	abnormal dryness, eg of the skin, mouth, eyes, etc
xerostomia	excessive dryness of the mouth as a result of insufficient secretions

Zz

zo-, zoo-
denoting animals
combining form
From Greek ***zōion*** = living thing, animal

zoograft	a piece of animal tissue grafted onto a human
zoonosis	a disease of animals which can be transmitted to humans, such as rabies
zoophilia	sexual attraction towards animals
zoopsia	a form of mental delusion in which one sees animals

zona
a zona pellucida; shingles (herpes zoster)
noun
From Latin ***zona***, from Greek ***zōnē*** = belt, girdle, shingles
Plural form **zonae**

zona pellucida   a thick, transparent membrane around the mature ovum

zonula
a small zone or band
noun
From Latin **zonula** = little girdle, from **zona**, from Greek **zōnē** = belt, girdle, shingles
Plural form **zonulae**

zoo- see ▸ zo-, zoo-

-zoon
denoting an animal or a free-moving cell
combining form
From Greek **zōion** = living thing, animal
Plural form **-zoa** (or **-zoons**)

ento**zoon**	an animal that lives as a parasite within the body of its host
epi**zoon**	an animal that lives on the surface of another animal, whether parasitically or commensally
spermato**zoon**	a male sex cell, any of the millions contained in semen

zyg-, zygo-
denoting yoke, union or pair
combining form
From Greek **zygon** = yoke

zygapophysis	any of the articulations that link the vertebrae
zygotene	the second stage of the first phase of meiosis, in which the chromosomes form pairs

zygoma
the arch formed by the malar bone and the zygomatic process of the temporal bone of the skull
noun
From Greek **zygōma**, genitive **zygōmatos** = bolt, bar, zygomatic arch, from **zygon** = yoke
Plural form **zygomata** (or **zygomas**)

zygomatic
relating to or in the region of the ▸ **zygoma**
adjective
From Greek **zygōma**, genitive **zygōmatos** = bolt, bar, zygomatic arch, from **zygon** = yoke

zygomatic bone   the cheekbone

zygomatic process a projection of the temporal bone of the skull

zygote

the product of the union of two gametes; the individual developing from the product of the union of two gametes

noun

From Greek ***zygōtos*** = yoked, from ***zygon*** = yoke

◆ Related words **zygotic** *adj* ▸ relating to a zygote or the process of forming a zygote; existing as a zygote

-zygous

denoting a zygotic structure of the specified kind

combining form

From Greek ***zygon*** = yoke

hemi**zygous**	having only one representative of a gene or chromosome, as male mammals, which have only one X-chromosome
hetero**zygous**	having two different alleles of a gene
homo**zygous**	having two identical alleles of a gene

zym-, zymo-

denoting fermentation; denoting enzyme

combining form

From Greek ***zymē*** = leaven

zymogen	an inert precursor of many active proteins and degradative enzymes
zymolysis	the action of enzymes in fermentation

Latin and Greek grammar

CASE ENDINGS

Latin and Greek are inflecting languages. That means that relationships between the various words in a sentence are shown by changes in the form of each word, usually by alteration of its ending. English has a very basic system of inflections:

- you generally add -s to the singular of a noun to form the plural: dog → dog**s**
- you add -'s to the singular of a noun to form the possessive singular: dog → dog**'s**
- you add -s' to the singular of a noun to form the possessive plural: dog → dogs**'**

Latin and Greek simply take this system of modifying endings a lot further. Latin nouns have six forms or 'cases' in the singular and six in the plural, while Greek nouns have five in the singular and five in the plural.

These cases are as follows:

1. the **nominative** case shows that the noun is the subject of the sentence, as in *The man was reading a book*
2. the **vocative** case is used for addressing someone or something directly, as in *Can I help you, madam?*
3. the **accusative** case shows that the noun is the direct object of the sentence, as in *The man was reading a book*
4. the **genitive** case indicates possession, as in *Is that the man's book?* or *What's the title of the book?*
5. the **dative** case shows that the noun is the indirect object of the sentence, as in *She handed the book to the man* or *She bought a book for the man*
6. the **ablative** case is used mainly after prepositions such as those meaning 'by', 'with' or 'from'

The last, the ablative, is used only in Latin.

Latin and Greek nouns are always used in the nominative singular or plural in English, unless they occur in a phrase. In medicine, phrases are more commonly from Latin; some examples are given below.

Latin accusatives

Latin accusatives can be seen in the following words:

antepartum: formed from *ante*=before + *partum*, the accusative of *partus*=birth
postpartum: formed from *post*=after + *partum*, the accusative of *partus*=birth

Latin genitives

Latin genitives occur in the following phrases, for which a literal translation is given, with the nominative singular following in brackets:

> *sycosis **barbae*** =fig-like ulceration of the beard (***barba***)
> *tinea **barbae*** =worm of the beard (***barba***)
> *limbus **sclerae*** =edge of the sclera (***sclera***)
> *limen **nasi*** =threshold of the nose (***nasus***)
> *pons **Varolii*** =bridge of Varolius (from ***Varolius***, the Latinized form of the
>   surname of the Italian anatomist Constantio Varoli)
> *fornix **cerebri*** =arch of the brain (***cerebrum***)
> *mons **pubis*** =mountain of the pubic hair (***pubes***)
> *mons **Veneris*** =mountain of Venus (***Venus***)
> *planta **pedis*** =sole of the foot (***pes***)
> *porta **hepatis*** =gate of the liver (***hepar***)
> *rigor **mortis*** =stiffness of death (***mors***)

Latin ablatives

Latin ablatives can be seen in the following words:

> ***in utero***: formed from ***in*** =in + ***utero***, the ablative of ***uterus*** =womb
> ***in vitro***: formed from ***in*** =in + ***vitro***, the ablative of ***vitrum*** =glass
> ***in vivo***: formed from ***in*** =in + ***vivo***, the ablative of ***vivum*** =living thing

LATIN NOUNS

Latin nouns are divided into three genders: masculine, feminine or neuter.

Masculine nouns

Most masculine nouns end in **-us** in the nominative singular and form the nominative plural by changing the **-us** to **-i**, but a fairly large number retain the **-us** in the plural (which was pronounced with a long 'u' sound, to contrast it with the short 'u' sound of the singular).

humerus (upper arm, → *humeri* shoulder)	*saccus* (sack, bag) → *sacci*
limbus (edge) → *limbi*	*sartorius* (tailor's (muscle)) → *sartorii*
locus (place) → *loci*	*sulcus* (furrow) → *sulci*
naevus (mole, wart, spot) → *naevi*	*talus* (ankle, ankle bone, → *tali* heel)
nucleus (nut, kernel) → *nuclei*	*umbilicus* (navel) → *umbilici*
pilus (hair) → *pili*	*uterus* (womb) → *uteri*
radius (rod, spoke, ray, → *radii* radius)	*vagus* (wandering → *vagi* (nerve))
ramus (branch) → *rami*	*villus* (shaggy hair, tuft of → *villi* hair)
rectus (straight (muscle)) → *recti*	

but

fremitus (roaring) → *fremitus*	*hiatus* (opening, → *hiatus* aperture, cleft)

meatus (passage) → meatus   status (standing, position, → status
plexus (plaiting) → plexus   state, condition)

Note, however, that the plural of **sinus** is always **sinuses** in English.

Feminine nouns

Most feminine nouns end in -**a** in the nominative singular and form the nominative plural by changing the -**a** to -**ae**.

ala (wing) → alae
corona (wreath, crown)→ coronae
coxa (hip, hip bone) → coxae
crista (tuft, cockscomb, → cristae
crest)
decidua (falling-off → deciduae
(membrane))
fascia (band, bandage) → fasciae
fenestra (opening in a → fenestrae
wall, window)
fibula (clasp, buckle, pin) → fibulae
fistula (pipe, tube, fistula) → fistulae
fossa (ditch, trench) → fossae
fovea (small pit) → foveae
foveola (very small pit) → foveolae
galea (helmet) → galeae
gula (throat) → gulae
gutta (drop) → guttae
insula (island) → insulae
lacuna (pool, cavity, gap) → lacunae
lamina (thin plate or → laminae
layer)
linea (string, line) → lineae
macula (spot, mark, stain) → maculae
maxilla (jawbone, jaw) → maxillae

medulla (marrow) → medullae
mucosa (mucous → mucosae
(membrane))
planta (sole) → plantae
plica (fold) → plicae
porta (gate) → portae
ruga (wrinkle, crease, fold) → rugae
scapula (shoulder blade, → scapulae
shoulder)
seta (bristle) → setae
squama (scale) → squamae
stria (furrow, channel) → striae
tibia (shinbone, shin, → tibiae
pipe, flute)
tunica (tunic) → tunicae
ulna (elbow, arm) →ulnae
vena (blood vessel, vein, → venae
artery)
verruca (wart) → verrucae
vertebra (joint, vertebra) → vertebrae
vesica (bladder, blister) → vesicae
vita (life) → vitae
vulva (wrapper, covering, → vulvae
womb)
zonula (little girdle) → zonulae

There are some feminine nouns which end in -**us** in the nominative singular and retain the -**us** in the plural (which is pronounced with a long 'u' sound, to contrast it with the short 'u' sound of the singular). The commonest of these is:

manus → manus (hand)

Neuter nouns

Most neuter nouns end in -**um** in the nominative singular and form the nominative plural by changing the -**um** to -**a**:

antrum (cave) → antra

atrium (entrance hall) → atria

brachium (arm) → brachia

cerebrum (brain) → cerebra

cilium (eyelid) → cilia

hilum (trifle) → hila

ileum (groin, flank) → ilea

ilium (groin, flank) → ilia

infundibulum (funnel) → infundibula

labium (lip) → labia

milium (millet) → milia

ovum (egg) → ova

rectum (straight → recta (intestine))

reticulum (little net) → reticula

rostrum (beak, snout, → rostra muzzle)

sacrum (holy (bone)) → sacra

septum (fence, wall, → septa enclosure)

stratum (something → strata spread out)

Other groups of nouns

There are unfortunately many nouns, of all three genders, that do not fall into the above categories but form various subgroups. The most common of these in medical terminology are:

apex (top, tip) → apices

cortex (bark, covering) → cortices

pollex (thumb, big toe) → pollices

cervix (neck) → cervices

cicatrix (scar) → cicatrices

fornix (arch, vault) → fornices

radix (root) → radices

hallux (big toe) → halluces

foramen (opening) → foramina

limen (threshold) → limina

lumen (light, opening) → lumina

natis (buttock) → nates

pelvis (basin) → pelves

testis (witness, testicle) → testes

tussis (cough) → tusses

caput (head) → capita

occiput (back of the → occipita head)

cor (heart) → corda

corpus (body) → corpora

crus (leg) → crura

femur (thigh) → femora

viscus (internal organ) → viscera

genu (knee) → genua

mons (mountain) → montes

pons (bridge) → pontes

os (bone) → ossa

os (mouth) → ora

pes (foot) → pedes

rete (net) → retia

vas (vessel) → vasa

vertigo (turning round, → vertigines whirling round, dizziness, giddiness)

GREEK NOUNS

Greek nouns are also divided into three genders: masculine, feminine or neuter.

Masculine nouns

Most masculine nouns end in **-os** in the nominative singular and form the nominative plural by changing the **-os** to **-oi**. Greek masculine nouns ending in **-os** have usually entered English via Latin and so have the Latinized singular form of **-us** and plural form of **-i**.

> bronchus → bronchi [Greek *bronchos* (windpipe) → *bronchoi*]
> canthus → canthi [Greek *kanthos* (corner of the eye) → *kanthoi*]
> carpus → carpi [Greek *karpos* (wrist) → *karpoi*]
> gyrus → gyri [Greek *gyros* (ring, circle) → *gyroi*]
> isthmus → isthmi [Greek *isthmos* (neck, narrow passage) → *isthmoi*]
> oesophagus → oesophagi [Greek *oisophagos* (gullet) → *oisophagoi*]
> pylorus → pylori [Greek *pylōros* (gate-keeper, pylorus) → *pylōroi*]
> tarsus → tarsi [Greek *tarsos* (flat of the foot, ankle, edge of the eyelid
> and its lashes) → *tarsoi*]
> thalamus → thalami [Greek *thalamos* (inner room, bedroom) → *thalamoi*]
> thrombus → thrombi [Greek *thrombos* (lump, clot) → *thromboi*]
> thymus → thymi [Greek *thymos* (wart, thymus gland) → *thymoi*]

but note

> nephros → nephroi [Greek *nephros* (kidney) → *nephroi*]

Feminine nouns

Most feminine nouns end in either **-ē** or **-a** in the nominative singular and form the nominative plural by changing the **-ē** or **-a** ending to **-ai**. In English, Greek feminine nouns ending in **-ē** have usually entered the language via Latin and so have the Latinized singular form of **-a** and plural form of **-ae**. Greek feminine nouns ending in **-a** have also usually entered the language via Latin and so also have the Latinized plural form of **-ae**.

> chorda → chordae [Greek *chordē* (gut, gut string) → *chordai*]
> theca → thecae [Greek *thēkē* (case, sheath) → *thēkai*]
> zona → zonae [Greek *zōnē* (belt, girdle, shingles) → *zōnai*]
> glossa → glossae [Greek *glōssa* (tongue) → *glōssai*]
> pleura → pleurae [Greek *pleura* (rib, side) → *pleurai*]
> trachea → tracheae [Greek *tracheia* (rough (windpipe)) → *tracheiai*]

but note

> raphe → raphae [Greek *rhaphē* (seam, suture, stitching, sewing) →
> *rhaphai*]

Neuter nouns

Most neuter nouns end in **-on** in the nominative singular and form the nominative plural by changing the **-on** to **-a**. Most of these have entered English directly, not in a Latinized form:

> amnion (caul) → amnia
> chorion (membrane surrounding the embryo) → choria
> ganglion (encysted tumour on a tendon) → ganglia
> karyon (nut, kernel) → karya

Note, however, that the plural of **neuron** is always **neurons** in English.

Some of these Greek neuter nouns ending in **-on** in the nominative singular have, however, entered English via Latinized forms:

ischium → *ischia* [Greek *ischion* (hip joint) → *ischia*]

sternum → *sterna* [Greek *sternon* (chest, breast, breastbone) → *sterna*]

tympanum → *tympana* [Greek *tympanon* (kettledrum) → *tympana*]

Other groups of nouns

As with Latin there are many Greek nouns, of all three genders, that do not fall into the above categories but form various subgroups. Most have come via Latin and consequently have a Latinized spelling in English. The most common of these in medical terminology are:

thorax → *thoraces* [Greek *thōrax* (breastplate, trunk, chest) → *thōrakes*]

calyx → *calyces* [Greek *kalyx* (husk, cup of a flower) → *kalykes*]

coccyx → *coccyges* [Greek *kokkyx* (cuckoo, coccyx) → *kokkyges*]

phalanx → *phalanges* [Greek *phalanx* (troop formation, bone of finger or toe) → *phalanges*]

meninx → *meninges* [Greek *mēninx* (membrane) → *mēninges*]

salpinx → *salpinges* [Greek *salpinx* (trumpet) → *salpinges*]

larynx → *larynges* [Greek *larynx* (larynx) → *larynges*]

pharynx → *pharynges* [Greek *pharynx* (throat) → *pharynges*]

oedema → *oedemata* [Greek *oidēma* (swelling, tumour) → *oidēmata*]

carcinoma → *carcinomata* [Greek *karkinōma* (cancer) → *karkinōmata*]

soma → *somata* [Greek *sōma* (body) → *sōmata*]

stroma → *stromata* [Greek *strōma* (mattress, bed) → *strōmata*]

zygoma → *zygomata* [Greek *zygōma* (bolt, bar, zygomatic arch) → *zygōmata*]

stoma → *stomata* [Greek *stoma* (mouth) → *stomata*]

trauma → *traumata* [Greek *trauma* (wound) → *traumata*]

Greek nouns ending in **-sis** have entered English via Latin and form their plurals as in Latin:

cyesis → *cyeses* [Greek *kyēsis* (conception, pregnancy) → *kyēseis*]

ectasis → *ectases* [Greek *ektasis* (stretching out, extension) → *ektaseis*]

paresis → *pareses* [Greek *paresis* (releasing, relaxing) → *pareseis*]

sepsis → *sepses* [Greek *sēpsis* (putrefaction, decay) → *sēpseis*]

taxis → *taxes* [Greek *taxis* (arrangement, disposition, order, position) → *taxeis*]

ADJECTIVES

A Latin or Greek adjective agrees in case, number and gender with the noun to which it refers: if the noun is in the nominative, the adjective must also be in the nominative; if the noun is singular, the adjective must also be singular; and if the noun is masculine, the adjective must also be masculine. In many instances, this will mean that the noun and adjective have exactly the same endings, but it is not always so simple. Note that there are no Greek 'noun + adjective' phrases in medical terminology, so we can confine ourselves to Latin.

The commonest adjective types in Latin are:

> **-us, -a, -um**

for the masculine, feminine and neuter nominative singular respectively.
The corresponding plural forms are:

> **-i, -ae, -a**

Another common adjective type is:

> **-is, -is, -e**

for the masculine, feminine and neuter nominative singular respectively.
The corresponding plural forms are:

> **-es, -es, -ia**

Examples of where noun and adjective have the same ending (with a literal translation – see the main text for medical definitions):

> *lamina **propria*** (proper lamina)
> *linea **alba*** (white line)
> *locus **caeruleus*** (blue place)
> *macula **lutea*** (yellow spot)
> *medulla **oblongata*** (elongated medulla)
> *status **asthmaticus*** (asthmatic state)
> *status **epilepticus*** (epileptic state)
> *vena **cava*** (hollow vein)
> *zona **pellucida*** (transparent girdle)

but note the following (also given with a literal translation), where the adjective ending does not look the same as the noun's:

> ***dura** mater* (hard mother)
> *fovea **centralis*** (central depression)
> *genu **valgum*** (bow-legged knee)